MIGRAINE

JOURNAL

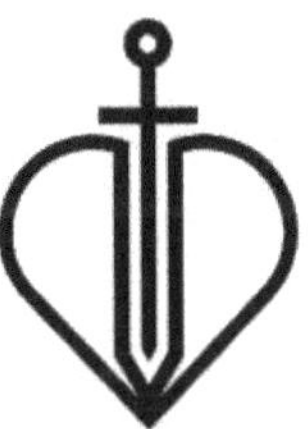

WELLNESS WARRIOR PRESS

ISBN: 978-1-990271-24-3

This journal belongs to...

____

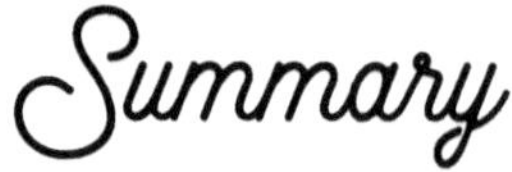

For each journal entry, return to this summary page and rate your overall pain / discomfort level (1 being no pain and 10 being unbearable)

Entry #	Date	Rating	Notes / Suspected Triggers
1			
2			
3			
4			
5			
6			
7			
8			
9			
10			
11			
12			
13			
14			
15			
16			
17			
18			
19			
20			
21			
22			
23			
24			
25			
26			
27			
28			
29			
30			

Summary – continued

For each journal entry, return to this summary page and rate your overall pain / discomfort level (1 being no pain and 10 being unbearable)

Entry #	Date	Rating	Notes / Suspected Triggers
31			
32			
33			
34			
35			
36			
37			
38			
39			
40			
41			
42			
43			
44			
45			
46			
47			
48			
49			
50			
51			
52			
53			
54			
55			
56			
57			
58			
59			
60			

My Calendar

	January	February	March	April	May	June	July	August	September	October	November	December
1												
2												
3												
4												
5												
6												
7												
8												
9												
10												
11												
12												
13												
14												
15												
16												
17												
18												
19												
20												
21												
22												
23												
24												
25												
26												
27												
28												
29												
30												
31												

Calendar Legend

Create your own legend using colors or codes.

Additional Notes

Entry #1

Date:________ **M T W T F S S**

START: | END: | DURATION:

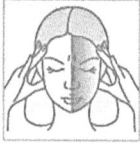

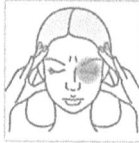

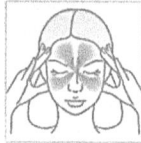

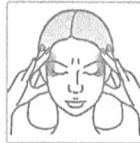

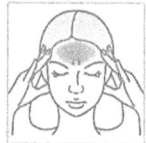

MIGRAINE CLUSTER SINUS TMJ TENSION

PAIN LEVEL

1	2	3	4	5	6	7	8	9	10

Not too bad. *Well, I'm not enjoying this.* *Make it stop!*

DETAILED DESCRIPTION

☐ Constant ☐ Squeezing ☐ Throbbing ☐ Pounding
☐ Dull aching ☐ Burning ☐ Sharp ☐ Debilitating

Other:________________________________

ONSET

☐ Slow ☐ Average ☐ Rapid ☐ Sudden

WHERE DOES IT HURT, EXACTLY?

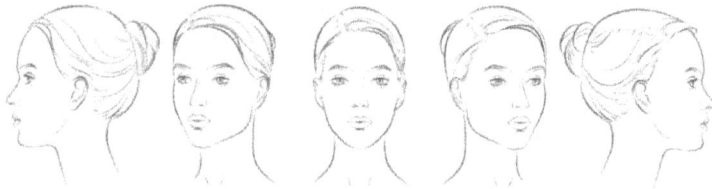

OTHER SYMPTOMS

☐ Lightheaded ☐ Dizziness ☐ Confusion
☐ Light sensitivity ☐ Sound sensitivity ☐ Auras
☐ Muscle stiffness ☐ Muscle burning ☐ Muscle aches

HOW ARE YOU FEELING OVERALL?

Mood	1	2	3	4	5	6	7	8	9	10
Energy levels	1	2	3	4	5	6	7	8	9	10
Mental clarity	1	2	3	4	5	6	7	8	9	10

Feeling sick?

☐ Nope!
☐ Yes...

☐ Nausea ☐ Diarrhea ☐ Vomiting ☐ Sore throat
☐ Congestion ☐ Coughing ☐ Chills ☐ Fever

Other symptoms: ________________________________

LAST NIGHT'S SLEEP

Hours of Sleep: ______________ Sleep Quality: ① ② ③ ④ ⑤

WEATHER

☐ Hot ☐ Mild ☐ Cold BM Pressure: _______

☐ Dry ☐ Humid ☐ Wet Allergen Levels: _______

☐ Sunny ☐ Cloudy

STRESS LEVELS

None	Low	Medium	High	Max	@$#%!

FOOD / DRINKS + NON-RELIEF MEDICATION / SUPPLEMENTS

item / meal	*time*	*meds / supplements*	*dose*	*time*

How many drinks?

water	① ② ③ ④ ⑤ ⑥ ⑦ ⑧ ⑨ ⑩
caffeine	① ② ③ ④ ⑤ ⑥ ⑦ ⑧ ⑨ ⑩
alcohol	① ② ③ ④ ⑤ ⑥ ⑦ ⑧ ⑨ ⑩

HORMONES

☐ Menstruating ☐ Menopause ☐ PMS ☐ N/A | other

COMPUTER USE / READING

☐ None ☐ Some ☐ A lot Total time: ☐

☐ Sitting ☐ Standing ☐ Mixture Breaks every: ☐

PHYSICAL ACTIVITY

☐ None ☐ Minimal ☐ Some ☐ Sweatin' ☐ I'm beat

DETAILS: ____

RELIEF MEASURES

☐ Medication ☐ Massage ☐ Sleep ☐ Exercise

☐ Water ☐ Cold/Ice ☐ Heat/Bath ☐ Other

DETAILS: ____

DID IT WORK? ☐ Nope ☐ A bit ☐ Mostly ☐ 100%

Notes

Entry #2

Date:________ M T W T F S S

START:		END:		DURATION:	

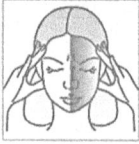

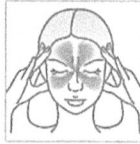

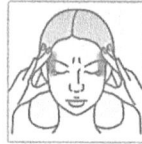

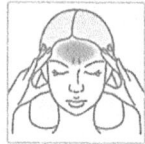

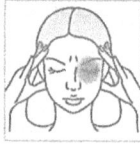

MIGRAINE CLUSTER SINUS TMJ TENSION

PAIN LEVEL

1	2	3	4	5	6	7	8	9	10

Not too bad. *Well, I'm not enjoying this.* *Make it stop!*

DETAILED DESCRIPTION

☐ Constant ☐ Squeezing ☐ Throbbing ☐ Pounding
☐ Dull aching ☐ Burning ☐ Sharp ☐ Debilitating

Other:______________________________

ONSET

☐ Slow ☐ Average ☐ Rapid ☐ Sudden

WHERE DOES IT HURT, EXACTLY?

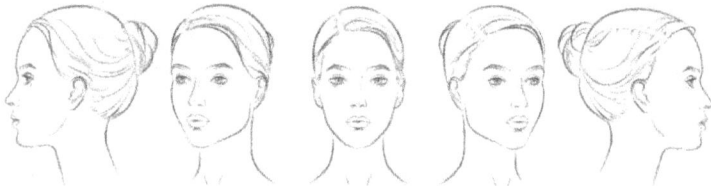

OTHER SYMPTOMS

☐ Lightheaded ☐ Dizziness ☐ Confusion
☐ Light sensitivity ☐ Sound sensitivity ☐ Auras
☐ Muscle stiffness ☐ Muscle burning ☐ Muscle aches

HOW ARE YOU FEELING OVERALL?

		Feeling sick?
Mood	① ② ③ ④ ⑤ ⑥ ⑦ ⑧ ⑨ ⑩	☐ Nope!
Energy levels	① ② ③ ④ ⑤ ⑥ ⑦ ⑧ ⑨ ⑩	☐ Yes...
Mental clarity	① ② ③ ④ ⑤ ⑥ ⑦ ⑧ ⑨ ⑩	

☐ Nausea ☐ Diarrhea ☐ Vomiting ☐ Sore throat
☐ Congestion ☐ Coughing ☐ Chills ☐ Fever

Other symptoms: ______________________________

LAST NIGHT'S SLEEP

Hours of Sleep: ____________ Sleep Quality: ① ② ③ ④ ⑤

WEATHER

☐ Hot ☐ Mild ☐ Cold BM Pressure: ______

☐ Dry ☐ Humid ☐ Wet Allergen Levels: ______

☐ Sunny ☐ Cloudy

STRESS LEVELS

None	Low	Medium	High	Max	@$#%!

FOOD / DRINKS + NON-RELIEF MEDICATION / SUPPLEMENTS

item / meal	*time*	*meds / supplements*	*dose*	*time*

How many drinks?

water	① ② ③ ④ ⑤ ⑥ ⑦ ⑧ ⑨ ⑩
caffeine	① ② ③ ④ ⑤ ⑥ ⑦ ⑧ ⑨ ⑩
alcohol	① ② ③ ④ ⑤ ⑥ ⑦ ⑧ ⑨ ⑩

HORMONES

☐ Menstruating ☐ Menopause ☐ PMS ☐ N/A | other

COMPUTER USE / READING

☐ None ☐ Some ☐ A lot Total time:

☐ Sitting ☐ Standing ☐ Mixture Breaks every:

PHYSICAL ACTIVITY

☐ None ☐ Minimal ☐ Some ☐ Sweatin' ☐ I'm beat

DETAILS: ______________________________

RELIEF MEASURES

☐ Medication ☐ Massage ☐ Sleep ☐ Exercise

☐ Water ☐ Cold/Ice ☐ Heat/Bath ☐ Other

DETAILS: ______________________________

DID IT WORK? ☐ Nope ☐ A bit ☐ Mostly ☐ 100%

Notes

Entry #3

Date:_________ M T W T F S S

START:		END:		DURATION:	

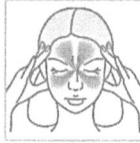

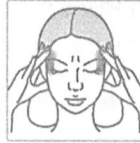

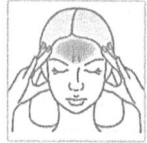

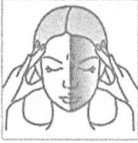

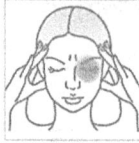

MIGRAINE CLUSTER SINUS TMJ TENSION

PAIN LEVEL

1	2	3	4	5	6	7	8	9	10

Not too bad. *Well, I'm not enjoying this.* *Make it stop!*

DETAILED DESCRIPTION

☐ Constant ☐ Squeezing ☐ Throbbing ☐ Pounding
☐ Dull aching ☐ Burning ☐ Sharp ☐ Debilitating

Other:____________________

ONSET

☐ Slow ☐ Average ☐ Rapid ☐ Sudden

WHERE DOES IT HURT, EXACTLY?

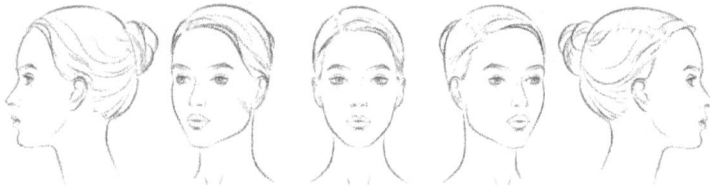

OTHER SYMPTOMS

☐ Lightheaded ☐ Dizziness ☐ Confusion
☐ Light sensitivity ☐ Sound sensitivity ☐ Auras
☐ Muscle stiffness ☐ Muscle burning ☐ Muscle aches

HOW ARE YOU FEELING OVERALL?

Mood	1	2	3	4	5	6	7	8	9	10
Energy levels	1	2	3	4	5	6	7	8	9	10
Mental clarity	1	2	3	4	5	6	7	8	9	10

Feeling sick?

☐ Nope!
☐ Yes...

☐ Nausea ☐ Diarrhea ☐ Vomiting ☐ Sore throat
☐ Congestion ☐ Coughing ☐ Chills ☐ Fever

Other symptoms: ____________________

LAST NIGHT'S SLEEP

Hours of Sleep: ____________ Sleep Quality: ① ② ③ ④ ⑤

WEATHER

☐ Hot ☐ Mild ☐ Cold BM Pressure: ______

☐ Dry ☐ Humid ☐ Wet Allergen Levels: ______

☐ Sunny ☐ Cloudy

STRESS LEVELS

None	Low	Medium	High	Max	@$#%!

FOOD / DRINKS + NON-RELIEF MEDICATION / SUPPLEMENTS

item / meal	*time*	*meds / supplements*	*dose*	*time*

How many drinks?

water	1	2	3	4	5	6	7	8	9	10
caffeine	1	2	3	4	5	6	7	8	9	10
alcohol	1	2	3	4	5	6	7	8	9	10

HORMONES

☐ Menstruating ☐ Menopause ☐ PMS ☐ N/A | other

COMPUTER USE / READING

☐ None ☐ Some ☐ A lot Total time:

☐ Sitting ☐ Standing ☐ Mixture Breaks every:

PHYSICAL ACTIVITY

☐ None ☐ Minimal ☐ Some ☐ Sweatin' ☐ I'm beat

DETAILS: ______________________________

RELIEF MEASURES

☐ Medication ☐ Massage ☐ Sleep ☐ Exercise

☐ Water ☐ Cold/Ice ☐ Heat/Bath ☐ Other

DETAILS: ______________________________

DID IT WORK? ☐ Nope ☐ A bit ☐ Mostly ☐ 100%

Notes

Entry #4

Date:________ M T W T F S S

START:		END:		DURATION:	

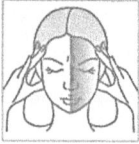

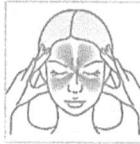

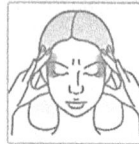

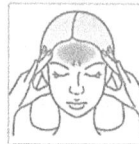

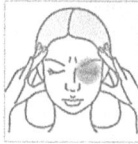

MIGRAINE CLUSTER SINUS TMJ TENSION

PAIN LEVEL

1	2	3	4	5	6	7	8	9	10

Not too bad. *Well, I'm not enjoying this.* *Make it stop!*

DETAILED DESCRIPTION

☐ Constant ☐ Squeezing ☐ Throbbing ☐ Pounding
☐ Dull aching ☐ Burning ☐ Sharp ☐ Debilitating

Other:____

ONSET

☐ Slow ☐ Average ☐ Rapid ☐ Sudden

WHERE DOES IT HURT, EXACTLY?

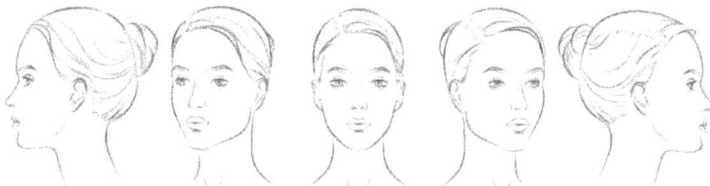

OTHER SYMPTOMS

☐ Lightheaded ☐ Dizziness ☐ Confusion
☐ Light sensitivity ☐ Sound sensitivity ☐ Auras
☐ Muscle stiffness ☐ Muscle burning ☐ Muscle aches

HOW ARE YOU FEELING OVERALL?

Mood	1	2	3	4	5	6	7	8	9	10
Energy levels	1	2	3	4	5	6	7	8	9	10
Mental clarity	1	2	3	4	5	6	7	8	9	10

Feeling sick?

☐ Nope!
☐ Yes...

☐ Nausea ☐ Diarrhea ☐ Vomiting ☐ Sore throat
☐ Congestion ☐ Coughing ☐ Chills ☐ Fever

Other symptoms: ________________________________

LAST NIGHT'S SLEEP

Hours of Sleep: ____________ Sleep Quality: (1) (2) (3) (4) (5)

WEATHER

☐ Hot ☐ Mild ☐ Cold BM Pressure: ______

☐ Dry ☐ Humid ☐ Wet Allergen Levels: ______

☐ Sunny ☐ Cloudy

STRESS LEVELS

None	Low	Medium	High	Max	@$#%!

FOOD / DRINKS + NON-RELIEF MEDICATION / SUPPLEMENTS

item / meal	*time*	*meds / supplements*	*dose*	*time*

How many drinks?

water	1	2	3	4	5	6	7	8	9	10
caffeine	1	2	3	4	5	6	7	8	9	10
alcohol	1	2	3	4	5	6	7	8	9	10

HORMONES

☐ Menstruating ☐ Menopause ☐ PMS ☐ N/A | other

COMPUTER USE / READING

☐ None ☐ Some ☐ A lot Total time:

☐ Sitting ☐ Standing ☐ Mixture Breaks every:

PHYSICAL ACTIVITY

☐ None ☐ Minimal ☐ Some ☐ Sweatin' ☐ I'm beat

DETAILS: ______________________________

RELIEF MEASURES

☐ Medication ☐ Massage ☐ Sleep ☐ Exercise

☐ Water ☐ Cold/Ice ☐ Heat/Bath ☐ Other

DETAILS: ______________________________

DID IT WORK? ☐ Nope ☐ A bit ☐ Mostly ☐ 100%

Notes

Entry #5

Date:________ M T W T F S S

START:		END:		DURATION:	

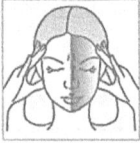

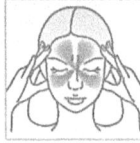

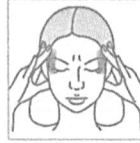

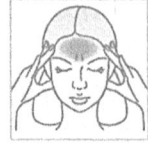

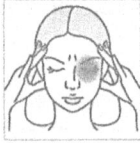

MIGRAINE CLUSTER SINUS TMJ TENSION

PAIN LEVEL

1	2	3	4	5	6	7	8	9	10

Not too bad. *Well, I'm not enjoying this.* *Make it stop!*

DETAILED DESCRIPTION

☐ Constant ☐ Squeezing ☐ Throbbing ☐ Pounding
☐ Dull aching ☐ Burning ☐ Sharp ☐ Debilitating

Other:______________________________

ONSET

☐ Slow ☐ Average ☐ Rapid ☐ Sudden

WHERE DOES IT HURT, EXACTLY?

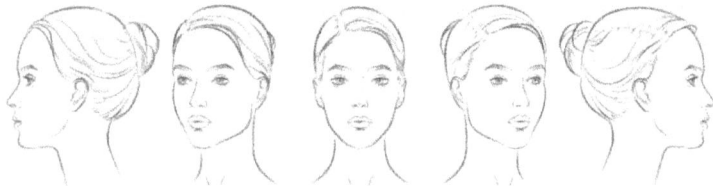

OTHER SYMPTOMS

☐ Lightheaded ☐ Dizziness ☐ Confusion
☐ Light sensitivity ☐ Sound sensitivity ☐ Auras
☐ Muscle stiffness ☐ Muscle burning ☐ Muscle aches

HOW ARE YOU FEELING OVERALL?

Mood	1	2	3	4	5	6	7	8	9	10
Energy levels	1	2	3	4	5	6	7	8	9	10
Mental clarity	1	2	3	4	5	6	7	8	9	10

Feeling sick?

☐ Nope!
☐ Yes...

☐ Nausea ☐ Diarrhea ☐ Vomiting ☐ Sore throat
☐ Congestion ☐ Coughing ☐ Chills ☐ Fever

Other symptoms: ______________________________

LAST NIGHT'S SLEEP

Hours of Sleep: ____________ Sleep Quality: ① ② ③ ④ ⑤

WEATHER

☐ Hot ☐ Mild ☐ Cold BM Pressure: ______

☐ Dry ☐ Humid ☐ Wet Allergen Levels: ______

☐ Sunny ☐ Cloudy

STRESS LEVELS

None	Low	Medium	High	Max	@$#%!

FOOD / DRINKS + NON-RELIEF MEDICATION / SUPPLEMENTS

item / meal	*time*	*meds / supplements*	*dose*	*time*

How many drinks?

water	① ② ③ ④ ⑤ ⑥ ⑦ ⑧ ⑨ ⑩
caffeine	① ② ③ ④ ⑤ ⑥ ⑦ ⑧ ⑨ ⑩
alcohol	① ② ③ ④ ⑤ ⑥ ⑦ ⑧ ⑨ ⑩

HORMONES

☐ Menstruating ☐ Menopause ☐ PMS ☐ N/A | other

COMPUTER USE / READING

☐ None ☐ Some ☐ A lot Total time: ______

☐ Sitting ☐ Standing ☐ Mixture Breaks every: ______

PHYSICAL ACTIVITY

☐ None ☐ Minimal ☐ Some ☐ Sweatin' ☐ I'm beat

DETAILS: ________________________________

RELIEF MEASURES

☐ Medication ☐ Massage ☐ Sleep ☐ Exercise

☐ Water ☐ Cold/Ice ☐ Heat/Bath ☐ Other

DETAILS: ________________________________

DID IT WORK? ☐ Nope ☐ A bit ☐ Mostly ☐ 100%

Notes

Entry #6

Date:________ **M T W T F S S**

START:		END:		DURATION:	

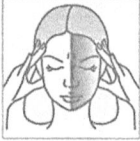

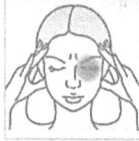

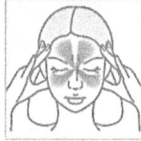

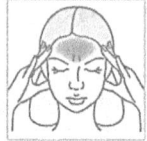

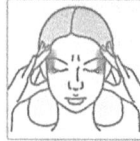

MIGRAINE CLUSTER SINUS TMJ TENSION

PAIN LEVEL

1	2	3	4	5	6	7	8	9	10

Not too bad. *Well, I'm not enjoying this.* *Make it stop!*

DETAILED DESCRIPTION

☐ Constant ☐ Squeezing ☐ Throbbing ☐ Pounding
☐ Dull aching ☐ Burning ☐ Sharp ☐ Debilitating

Other:________________________________

ONSET

☐ Slow ☐ Average ☐ Rapid ☐ Sudden

WHERE DOES IT HURT, EXACTLY?

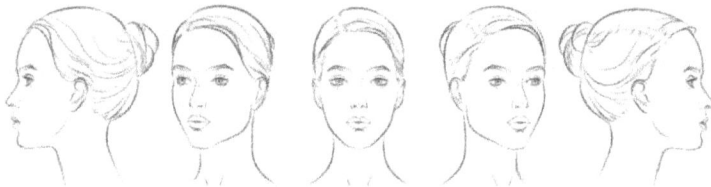

OTHER SYMPTOMS

☐ Lightheaded ☐ Dizziness ☐ Confusion
☐ Light sensitivity ☐ Sound sensitivity ☐ Auras
☐ Muscle stiffness ☐ Muscle burning ☐ Muscle aches

HOW ARE YOU FEELING OVERALL?

Mood	1	2	3	4	5	6	7	8	9	10
Energy levels	1	2	3	4	5	6	7	8	9	10
Mental clarity	1	2	3	4	5	6	7	8	9	10

Feeling sick?

☐ Nope!
☐ Yes…

☐ Nausea ☐ Diarrhea ☐ Vomiting ☐ Sore throat
☐ Congestion ☐ Coughing ☐ Chills ☐ Fever

Other symptoms: ________________________________

LAST NIGHT'S SLEEP

Hours of Sleep: ____________ Sleep Quality: ① ② ③ ④ ⑤

WEATHER

☐ Hot ☐ Mild ☐ Cold BM Pressure: ______

☐ Dry ☐ Humid ☐ Wet Allergen Levels: ______

☐ Sunny ☐ Cloudy

STRESS LEVELS

None	Low	Medium	High	Max	@$#%!

FOOD / DRINKS + NON-RELIEF MEDICATION / SUPPLEMENTS

item / meal	*time*	*meds / supplements*	*dose*	*time*

How many drinks?

water	① ② ③ ④ ⑤ ⑥ ⑦ ⑧ ⑨ ⑩
caffeine	① ② ③ ④ ⑤ ⑥ ⑦ ⑧ ⑨ ⑩
alcohol	① ② ③ ④ ⑤ ⑥ ⑦ ⑧ ⑨ ⑩

HORMONES

☐ Menstruating ☐ Menopause ☐ PMS ☐ N/A | other

COMPUTER USE / READING

☐ None ☐ Some ☐ A lot Total time: ______

☐ Sitting ☐ Standing ☐ Mixture Breaks every: ______

PHYSICAL ACTIVITY

☐ None ☐ Minimal ☐ Some ☐ Sweatin' ☐ I'm beat

DETAILS: ________________________________

RELIEF MEASURES

☐ Medication ☐ Massage ☐ Sleep ☐ Exercise

☐ Water ☐ Cold/Ice ☐ Heat/Bath ☐ Other

DETAILS: ________________________________

DID IT WORK? ☐ Nope ☐ A bit ☐ Mostly ☐ 100%

Notes

Entry #7

Date: ________ M T W T F S S

START:		END:		DURATION:	

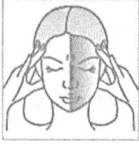

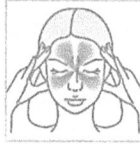

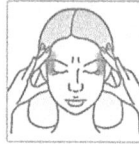

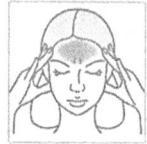

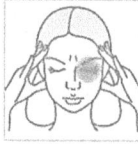

MIGRAINE CLUSTER SINUS TMJ TENSION

PAIN LEVEL

1	2	3	4	5	6	7	8	9	10

Not too bad. *Well, I'm not enjoying this.* *Make it stop!*

DETAILED DESCRIPTION

☐ Constant ☐ Squeezing ☐ Throbbing ☐ Pounding
☐ Dull aching ☐ Burning ☐ Sharp ☐ Debilitating

Other:____________________

ONSET

☐ Slow ☐ Average ☐ Rapid ☐ Sudden

WHERE DOES IT HURT, EXACTLY?

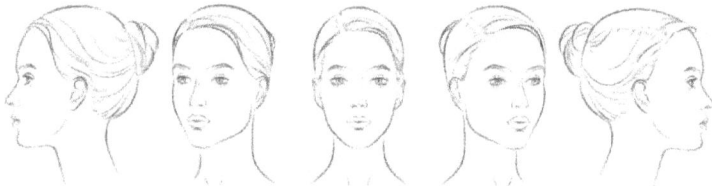

OTHER SYMPTOMS

☐ Lightheaded ☐ Dizziness ☐ Confusion
☐ Light sensitivity ☐ Sound sensitivity ☐ Auras
☐ Muscle stiffness ☐ Muscle burning ☐ Muscle aches

HOW ARE YOU FEELING OVERALL?

Mood	1	2	3	4	5	6	7	8	9	10
Energy levels	1	2	3	4	5	6	7	8	9	10
Mental clarity	1	2	3	4	5	6	7	8	9	10

Feeling sick?

☐ Nope!
☐ Yes...

☐ Nausea ☐ Diarrhea ☐ Vomiting ☐ Sore throat
☐ Congestion ☐ Coughing ☐ Chills ☐ Fever

Other symptoms: ____________________

LAST NIGHT'S SLEEP

Hours of Sleep: ____________ Sleep Quality: ① ② ③ ④ ⑤

WEATHER

☐ Hot ☐ Mild ☐ Cold BM Pressure: ______

☐ Dry ☐ Humid ☐ Wet Allergen Levels: ______

☐ Sunny ☐ Cloudy

STRESS LEVELS

None	Low	Medium	High	Max	@$#%!

FOOD / DRINKS + NON-RELIEF MEDICATION / SUPPLEMENTS

item / meal	*time*	*meds / supplements*	*dose*	*time*

How many drinks?

water →	① ② ③ ④ ⑤ ⑥ ⑦ ⑧ ⑨ ⑩
caffeine →	① ② ③ ④ ⑤ ⑥ ⑦ ⑧ ⑨ ⑩
alcohol →	① ② ③ ④ ⑤ ⑥ ⑦ ⑧ ⑨ ⑩

HORMONES

☐ Menstruating ☐ Menopause ☐ PMS ☐ N/A | other

COMPUTER USE / READING

☐ None ☐ Some ☐ A lot Total time: ______

☐ Sitting ☐ Standing ☐ Mixture Breaks every: ______

PHYSICAL ACTIVITY

☐ None ☐ Minimal ☐ Some ☐ Sweatin' ☐ I'm beat

DETAILS: ________________________________

RELIEF MEASURES

☐ Medication ☐ Massage ☐ Sleep ☐ Exercise

☐ Water ☐ Cold/Ice ☐ Heat/Bath ☐ Other

DETAILS: ________________________________

DID IT WORK? ☐ Nope ☐ A bit ☐ Mostly ☐ 100%

Notes

Entry #8

Date:________ M T W T F S S

START:		END:		DURATION:	

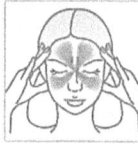

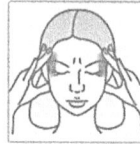

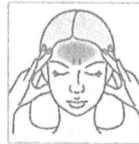

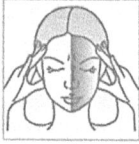

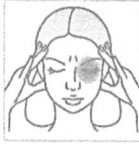

MIGRAINE CLUSTER SINUS TMJ TENSION

PAIN LEVEL

1	2	3	4	5	6	7	8	9	10

Not too bad. *Well, I'm not enjoying this.* *Make it stop!*

DETAILED DESCRIPTION

☐ Constant ☐ Squeezing ☐ Throbbing ☐ Pounding
☐ Dull aching ☐ Burning ☐ Sharp ☐ Debilitating

Other:____________________

ONSET

☐ Slow ☐ Average ☐ Rapid ☐ Sudden

WHERE DOES IT HURT, EXACTLY?

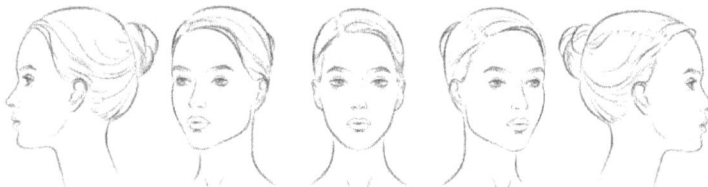

OTHER SYMPTOMS

☐ Lightheaded ☐ Dizziness ☐ Confusion
☐ Light sensitivity ☐ Sound sensitivity ☐ Auras
☐ Muscle stiffness ☐ Muscle burning ☐ Muscle aches

HOW ARE YOU FEELING OVERALL?

		Feeling sick?
Mood	① ② ③ ④ ⑤ ⑥ ⑦ ⑧ ⑨ ⑩	☐ Nope!
Energy levels	① ② ③ ④ ⑤ ⑥ ⑦ ⑧ ⑨ ⑩	☐ Yes...
Mental clarity	① ② ③ ④ ⑤ ⑥ ⑦ ⑧ ⑨ ⑩	

☐ Nausea ☐ Diarrhea ☐ Vomiting ☐ Sore throat
☐ Congestion ☐ Coughing ☐ Chills ☐ Fever

Other symptoms: ____________________

LAST NIGHT'S SLEEP

Hours of Sleep: ____________ Sleep Quality: ① ② ③ ④ ⑤

WEATHER

☐ Hot ☐ Mild ☐ Cold BM Pressure: ______

☐ Dry ☐ Humid ☐ Wet Allergen Levels: ______

☐ Sunny ☐ Cloudy

STRESS LEVELS

None	Low	Medium	High	Max	@$#%!

FOOD / DRINKS + NON-RELIEF MEDICATION / SUPPLEMENTS

item / meal	*time*	*meds / supplements*	*dose*	*time*

How many drinks?

water	① ② ③ ④ ⑤ ⑥ ⑦ ⑧ ⑨ ⑩
caffeine	① ② ③ ④ ⑤ ⑥ ⑦ ⑧ ⑨ ⑩
alcohol	① ② ③ ④ ⑤ ⑥ ⑦ ⑧ ⑨ ⑩

HORMONES

☐ Menstruating ☐ Menopause ☐ PMS ☐ N/A | other

COMPUTER USE / READING

☐ None ☐ Some ☐ A lot Total time:

☐ Sitting ☐ Standing ☐ Mixture Breaks every:

PHYSICAL ACTIVITY

☐ None ☐ Minimal ☐ Some ☐ Sweatin' ☐ I'm beat

DETAILS: ________________________________

RELIEF MEASURES

☐ Medication ☐ Massage ☐ Sleep ☐ Exercise

☐ Water ☐ Cold/Ice ☐ Heat/Bath ☐ Other

DETAILS: ________________________________

DID IT WORK? ☐ Nope ☐ A bit ☐ Mostly ☐ 100%

Notes

Entry #9

Date:________ M T W T F S S

START:		END:		DURATION:	

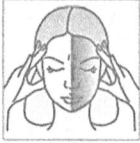

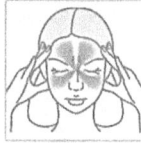

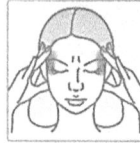

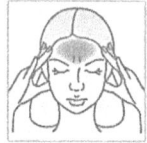

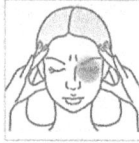

MIGRAINE CLUSTER SINUS TMJ TENSION

PAIN LEVEL

1	2	3	4	5	6	7	8	9	10

Not too bad. *Well, I'm not enjoying this.* *Make it stop!*

DETAILED DESCRIPTION

☐ Constant ☐ Squeezing ☐ Throbbing ☐ Pounding
☐ Dull aching ☐ Burning ☐ Sharp ☐ Debilitating

Other:___________________________

ONSET

☐ Slow ☐ Average ☐ Rapid ☐ Sudden

WHERE DOES IT HURT, EXACTLY?

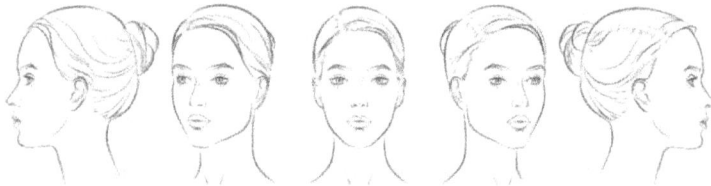

OTHER SYMPTOMS

☐ Lightheaded ☐ Dizziness ☐ Confusion
☐ Light sensitivity ☐ Sound sensitivity ☐ Auras
☐ Muscle stiffness ☐ Muscle burning ☐ Muscle aches

HOW ARE YOU FEELING OVERALL?

Mood	1	2	3	4	5	6	7	8	9	10
Energy levels	1	2	3	4	5	6	7	8	9	10
Mental clarity	1	2	3	4	5	6	7	8	9	10

Feeling sick?

☐ Nope!
☐ Yes...

☐ Nausea ☐ Diarrhea ☐ Vomiting ☐ Sore throat
☐ Congestion ☐ Coughing ☐ Chills ☐ Fever

Other symptoms: ___________________________

LAST NIGHT'S SLEEP

Hours of Sleep: ______________ Sleep Quality: ① ② ③ ④ ⑤

WEATHER

☐ Hot ☐ Mild ☐ Cold BM Pressure: ________

☐ Dry ☐ Humid ☐ Wet Allergen Levels: ________

☐ Sunny ☐ Cloudy

STRESS LEVELS

None	Low	Medium	High	Max	@$#%!

FOOD / DRINKS + NON-RELIEF MEDICATION / SUPPLEMENTS

item / meal	*time*	*meds / supplements*	*dose*	*time*

How many drinks?

water	① ② ③ ④ ⑤ ⑥ ⑦ ⑧ ⑨ ⑩
caffeine	① ② ③ ④ ⑤ ⑥ ⑦ ⑧ ⑨ ⑩
alcohol	① ② ③ ④ ⑤ ⑥ ⑦ ⑧ ⑨ ⑩

HORMONES

☐ Menstruating ☐ Menopause ☐ PMS ☐ N/A | other

COMPUTER USE / READING

☐ None ☐ Some ☐ A lot Total time: ________

☐ Sitting ☐ Standing ☐ Mixture Breaks every: ________

PHYSICAL ACTIVITY

☐ None ☐ Minimal ☐ Some ☐ Sweatin' ☐ I'm beat

DETAILS: ____

RELIEF MEASURES

☐ Medication ☐ Massage ☐ Sleep ☐ Exercise

☐ Water ☐ Cold/Ice ☐ Heat/Bath ☐ Other

DETAILS: ____

DID IT WORK? ☐ Nope ☐ A bit ☐ Mostly ☐ 100%

Notes

Entry #10

Date: ________ M T W T F S S

START:		END:		DURATION:	

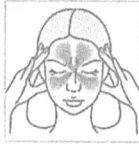

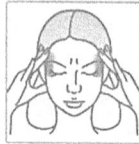

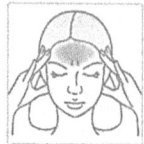

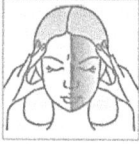

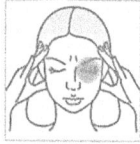

MIGRAINE CLUSTER SINUS TMJ TENSION

PAIN LEVEL

1	2	3	4	5	6	7	8	9	10

Not too bad. *Well, I'm not enjoying this.* *Make it stop!*

DETAILED DESCRIPTION

☐ Constant ☐ Squeezing ☐ Throbbing ☐ Pounding
☐ Dull aching ☐ Burning ☐ Sharp ☐ Debilitating

Other:________________________________

ONSET

☐ Slow ☐ Average ☐ Rapid ☐ Sudden

WHERE DOES IT HURT, EXACTLY?

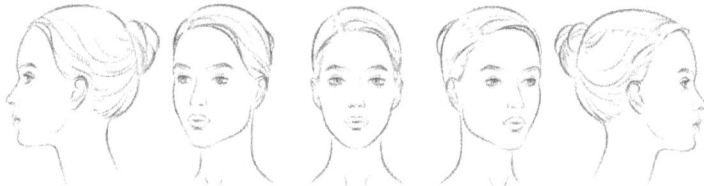

OTHER SYMPTOMS

☐ Lightheaded ☐ Dizziness ☐ Confusion
☐ Light sensitivity ☐ Sound sensitivity ☐ Auras
☐ Muscle stiffness ☐ Muscle burning ☐ Muscle aches

HOW ARE YOU FEELING OVERALL?

		Feeling sick?
Mood	① ② ③ ④ ⑤ ⑥ ⑦ ⑧ ⑨ ⑩	☐ Nope!
Energy levels	① ② ③ ④ ⑤ ⑥ ⑦ ⑧ ⑨ ⑩	☐ Yes...
Mental clarity	① ② ③ ④ ⑤ ⑥ ⑦ ⑧ ⑨ ⑩	

☐ Nausea ☐ Diarrhea ☐ Vomiting ☐ Sore throat
☐ Congestion ☐ Coughing ☐ Chills ☐ Fever

Other symptoms: ________________________________

LAST NIGHT'S SLEEP

Hours of Sleep: ____________ Sleep Quality: ① ② ③ ④ ⑤

WEATHER

☐ Hot ☐ Mild ☐ Cold BM Pressure: ______
☐ Dry ☐ Humid ☐ Wet Allergen Levels: ______
☐ Sunny ☐ Cloudy

STRESS LEVELS

None	Low	Medium	High	Max	@$#%!

FOOD / DRINKS + NON-RELIEF MEDICATION / SUPPLEMENTS

item / meal	*time*	*meds / supplements*	*dose*	*time*

How many drinks?

water	① ② ③ ④ ⑤ ⑥ ⑦ ⑧ ⑨ ⑩
caffeine	① ② ③ ④ ⑤ ⑥ ⑦ ⑧ ⑨ ⑩
alcohol	① ② ③ ④ ⑤ ⑥ ⑦ ⑧ ⑨ ⑩

HORMONES

☐ Menstruating ☐ Menopause ☐ PMS ☐ N/A | other

COMPUTER USE / READING

☐ None ☐ Some ☐ A lot Total time:
☐ Sitting ☐ Standing ☐ Mixture Breaks every:

PHYSICAL ACTIVITY

☐ None ☐ Minimal ☐ Some ☐ Sweatin' ☐ I'm beat

DETAILS: ____________________

RELIEF MEASURES

☐ Medication ☐ Massage ☐ Sleep ☐ Exercise
☐ Water ☐ Cold/Ice ☐ Heat/Bath ☐ Other

DETAILS: ____________________

DID IT WORK? ☐ Nope ☐ A bit ☐ Mostly ☐ 100%

Notes

Entry #11

Date:________ M T W T F S S

START:		END:		DURATION:	

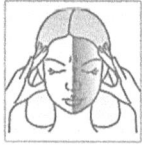

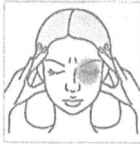

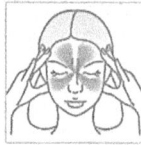

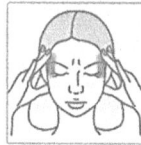

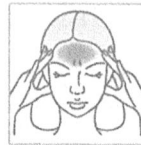

MIGRAINE CLUSTER SINUS TMJ TENSION

PAIN LEVEL

1	2	3	4	5	6	7	8	9	10

Not too bad. *Well, I'm not enjoying this.* *Make it stop!*

DETAILED DESCRIPTION

☐ Constant ☐ Squeezing ☐ Throbbing ☐ Pounding
☐ Dull aching ☐ Burning ☐ Sharp ☐ Debilitating

Other:______________________________

ONSET

☐ Slow ☐ Average ☐ Rapid ☐ Sudden

WHERE DOES IT HURT, EXACTLY?

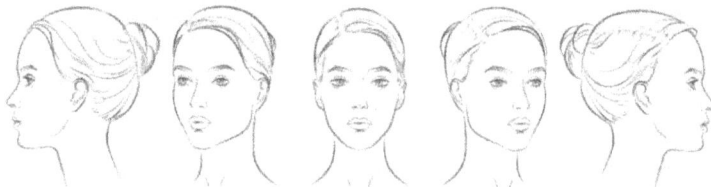

OTHER SYMPTOMS

☐ Lightheaded ☐ Dizziness ☐ Confusion
☐ Light sensitivity ☐ Sound sensitivity ☐ Auras
☐ Muscle stiffness ☐ Muscle burning ☐ Muscle aches

HOW ARE YOU FEELING OVERALL?

Mood	1	2	3	4	5	6	7	8	9	10
Energy levels	1	2	3	4	5	6	7	8	9	10
Mental clarity	1	2	3	4	5	6	7	8	9	10

Feeling sick?

☐ Nope!
☐ Yes...

☐ Nausea ☐ Diarrhea ☐ Vomiting ☐ Sore throat
☐ Congestion ☐ Coughing ☐ Chills ☐ Fever

Other symptoms: ______________________________

LAST NIGHT'S SLEEP

Hours of Sleep: ____________ Sleep Quality: ① ② ③ ④ ⑤

WEATHER

☐ Hot ☐ Mild ☐ Cold BM Pressure: ______

☐ Dry ☐ Humid ☐ Wet Allergen Levels: ______

☐ Sunny ☐ Cloudy

STRESS LEVELS

None	Low	Medium	High	Max	@$#%!

FOOD / DRINKS + NON-RELIEF MEDICATION / SUPPLEMENTS

item / meal	*time*	*meds / supplements*	*dose*	*time*

How many drinks?

water	1	2	3	4	5	6	7	8	9	10
caffeine	1	2	3	4	5	6	7	8	9	10
alcohol	1	2	3	4	5	6	7	8	9	10

HORMONES

☐ Menstruating ☐ Menopause ☐ PMS ☐ N/A | other

COMPUTER USE / READING

☐ None ☐ Some ☐ A lot Total time:

☐ Sitting ☐ Standing ☐ Mixture Breaks every:

PHYSICAL ACTIVITY

☐ None ☐ Minimal ☐ Some ☐ Sweatin' ☐ I'm beat

DETAILS: ______________________________

RELIEF MEASURES

☐ Medication ☐ Massage ☐ Sleep ☐ Exercise

☐ Water ☐ Cold/Ice ☐ Heat/Bath ☐ Other

DETAILS: ______________________________

DID IT WORK? ☐ Nope ☐ A bit ☐ Mostly ☐ 100%

Notes

Entry #12

Date:________ M T W T F S S

START:		END:		DURATION:	

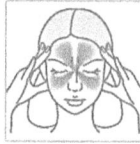

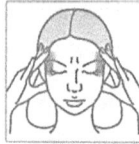

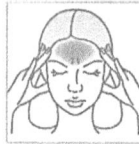

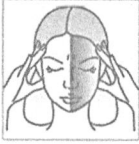

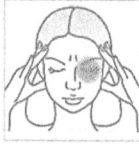

MIGRAINE CLUSTER SINUS TMJ TENSION

PAIN LEVEL

1	2	3	4	5	6	7	8	9	10

Not too bad. *Well, I'm not enjoying this.* *Make it stop!*

DETAILED DESCRIPTION

☐ Constant ☐ Squeezing ☐ Throbbing ☐ Pounding
☐ Dull aching ☐ Burning ☐ Sharp ☐ Debilitating

Other:____________________

ONSET

☐ Slow ☐ Average ☐ Rapid ☐ Sudden

WHERE DOES IT HURT, EXACTLY?

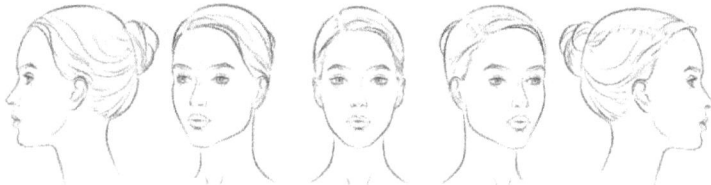

OTHER SYMPTOMS

☐ Lightheaded ☐ Dizziness ☐ Confusion
☐ Light sensitivity ☐ Sound sensitivity ☐ Auras
☐ Muscle stiffness ☐ Muscle burning ☐ Muscle aches

HOW ARE YOU FEELING OVERALL?

Mood	1	2	3	4	5	6	7	8	9	10
Energy levels	1	2	3	4	5	6	7	8	9	10
Mental clarity	1	2	3	4	5	6	7	8	9	10

Feeling sick?

☐ Nope!
☐ Yes...

☐ Nausea ☐ Diarrhea ☐ Vomiting ☐ Sore throat
☐ Congestion ☐ Coughing ☐ Chills ☐ Fever

Other symptoms:____________________

LAST NIGHT'S SLEEP

Hours of Sleep: ______________ Sleep Quality: ① ② ③ ④ ⑤

WEATHER

☐ Hot ☐ Mild ☐ Cold BM Pressure: _______
☐ Dry ☐ Humid ☐ Wet Allergen Levels: _______
☐ Sunny ☐ Cloudy

STRESS LEVELS

None	Low	Medium	High	Max	@$#%!

FOOD / DRINKS + NON-RELIEF MEDICATION / SUPPLEMENTS

item / meal	time	meds / supplements	dose	time

How many drinks?

water	① ② ③ ④ ⑤ ⑥ ⑦ ⑧ ⑨ ⑩
caffeine	① ② ③ ④ ⑤ ⑥ ⑦ ⑧ ⑨ ⑩
alcohol	① ② ③ ④ ⑤ ⑥ ⑦ ⑧ ⑨ ⑩

HORMONES

☐ Menstruating ☐ Menopause ☐ PMS ☐ N/A | other

COMPUTER USE / READING

☐ None ☐ Some ☐ A lot Total time:
☐ Sitting ☐ Standing ☐ Mixture Breaks every:

PHYSICAL ACTIVITY

☐ None ☐ Minimal ☐ Some ☐ Sweatin' ☐ I'm beat

DETAILS: ____

RELIEF MEASURES

☐ Medication ☐ Massage ☐ Sleep ☐ Exercise
☐ Water ☐ Cold/Ice ☐ Heat/Bath ☐ Other

DETAILS: ____

DID IT WORK? ☐ Nope ☐ A bit ☐ Mostly ☐ 100%

Notes

Entry #13

Date:_______

M T W T F S S

START:		END:		DURATION:	

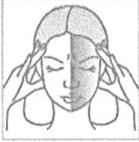

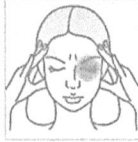

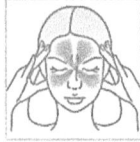

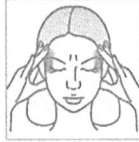

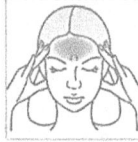

MIGRAINE CLUSTER SINUS TMJ TENSION

PAIN LEVEL

1	2	3	4	5	6	7	8	9	10

Not too bad. *Well, I'm not enjoying this.* *Make it stop!*

DETAILED DESCRIPTION

☐ Constant ☐ Squeezing ☐ Throbbing ☐ Pounding
☐ Dull aching ☐ Burning ☐ Sharp ☐ Debilitating

Other:_______________

ONSET

☐ Slow ☐ Average ☐ Rapid ☐ Sudden

WHERE DOES IT HURT, EXACTLY?

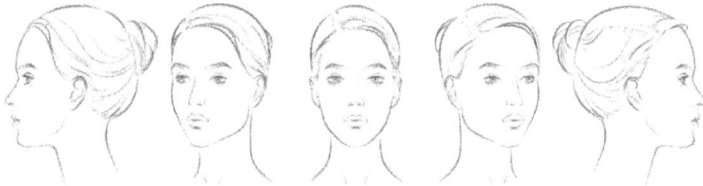

OTHER SYMPTOMS

☐ Lightheaded ☐ Dizziness ☐ Confusion
☐ Light sensitivity ☐ Sound sensitivity ☐ Auras
☐ Muscle stiffness ☐ Muscle burning ☐ Muscle aches

HOW ARE YOU FEELING OVERALL?

Mood	1	2	3	4	5	6	7	8	9	10
Energy levels	1	2	3	4	5	6	7	8	9	10
Mental clarity	1	2	3	4	5	6	7	8	9	10

Feeling sick?

☐ Nope!
☐ Yes...

☐ Nausea ☐ Diarrhea ☐ Vomiting ☐ Sore throat
☐ Congestion ☐ Coughing ☐ Chills ☐ Fever

Other symptoms: _______________

LAST NIGHT'S SLEEP

Hours of Sleep: ____________ Sleep Quality: ① ② ③ ④ ⑤

WEATHER

☐ Hot ☐ Mild ☐ Cold BM Pressure: ______

☐ Dry ☐ Humid ☐ Wet Allergen Levels: ______

☐ Sunny ☐ Cloudy

STRESS LEVELS

None	Low	Medium	High	Max	@$#%!

FOOD / DRINKS + NON-RELIEF MEDICATION / SUPPLEMENTS

item / meal	*time*	*meds / supplements*	*dose*	*time*

How many drinks?

water	① ② ③ ④ ⑤ ⑥ ⑦ ⑧ ⑨ ⑩
caffeine	① ② ③ ④ ⑤ ⑥ ⑦ ⑧ ⑨ ⑩
alcohol	① ② ③ ④ ⑤ ⑥ ⑦ ⑧ ⑨ ⑩

HORMONES

☐ Menstruating ☐ Menopause ☐ PMS ☐ N/A | other

COMPUTER USE / READING

☐ None ☐ Some ☐ A lot Total time:

☐ Sitting ☐ Standing ☐ Mixture Breaks every:

PHYSICAL ACTIVITY

☐ None ☐ Minimal ☐ Some ☐ Sweatin' ☐ I'm beat

DETAILS: ________________________________

RELIEF MEASURES

☐ Medication ☐ Massage ☐ Sleep ☐ Exercise

☐ Water ☐ Cold/Ice ☐ Heat/Bath ☐ Other

DETAILS: ________________________________

DID IT WORK? ☐ Nope ☐ A bit ☐ Mostly ☐ 100%

Notes

Entry #14

Date:________ M T W T F S S

START:		END:		DURATION:	

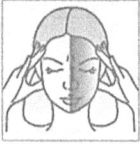

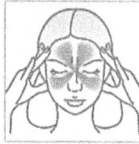

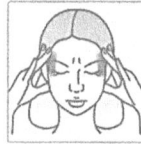

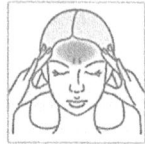

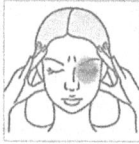

MIGRAINE CLUSTER SINUS TMJ TENSION

PAIN LEVEL

1	2	3	4	5	6	7	8	9	10

Not too bad. *Well, I'm not enjoying this.* *Make it stop!*

DETAILED DESCRIPTION

☐ Constant ☐ Squeezing ☐ Throbbing ☐ Pounding
☐ Dull aching ☐ Burning ☐ Sharp ☐ Debilitating

Other:______________________________

ONSET

☐ Slow ☐ Average ☐ Rapid ☐ Sudden

WHERE DOES IT HURT, EXACTLY?

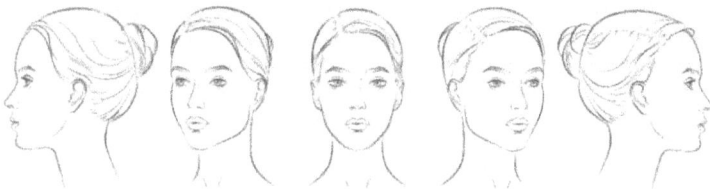

OTHER SYMPTOMS

☐ Lightheaded ☐ Dizziness ☐ Confusion
☐ Light sensitivity ☐ Sound sensitivity ☐ Auras
☐ Muscle stiffness ☐ Muscle burning ☐ Muscle aches

HOW ARE YOU FEELING OVERALL?

Mood	1	2	3	4	5	6	7	8	9	10
Energy levels	1	2	3	4	5	6	7	8	9	10
Mental clarity	1	2	3	4	5	6	7	8	9	10

Feeling sick?

☐ Nope!
☐ Yes...

☐ Nausea ☐ Diarrhea ☐ Vomiting ☐ Sore throat
☐ Congestion ☐ Coughing ☐ Chills ☐ Fever

Other symptoms: ______________________________

LAST NIGHT'S SLEEP

Hours of Sleep: ____________ Sleep Quality: ① ② ③ ④ ⑤

WEATHER

☐ Hot ☐ Mild ☐ Cold BM Pressure: _______

☐ Dry ☐ Humid ☐ Wet Allergen Levels: _______

☐ Sunny ☐ Cloudy

STRESS LEVELS

None	Low	Medium	High	Max	@$#%!

FOOD / DRINKS + NON-RELIEF MEDICATION / SUPPLEMENTS

item / meal	*time*	*meds / supplements*	*dose*	*time*

How many drinks?

water	① ② ③ ④ ⑤ ⑥ ⑦ ⑧ ⑨ ⑩
caffeine	① ② ③ ④ ⑤ ⑥ ⑦ ⑧ ⑨ ⑩
alcohol	① ② ③ ④ ⑤ ⑥ ⑦ ⑧ ⑨ ⑩

HORMONES

☐ Menstruating ☐ Menopause ☐ PMS ☐ N/A | other

COMPUTER USE / READING

☐ None ☐ Some ☐ A lot Total time: ☐

☐ Sitting ☐ Standing ☐ Mixture Breaks every: ☐

PHYSICAL ACTIVITY

☐ None ☐ Minimal ☐ Some ☐ Sweatin' ☐ I'm beat

DETAILS: ______________________________

RELIEF MEASURES

☐ Medication ☐ Massage ☐ Sleep ☐ Exercise

☐ Water ☐ Cold/Ice ☐ Heat/Bath ☐ Other

DETAILS: ______________________________

DID IT WORK? ☐ Nope ☐ A bit ☐ Mostly ☐ 100%

Notes

Entry #15

Date:________ M T W T F S S

START:		END:		DURATION:	

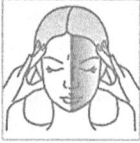

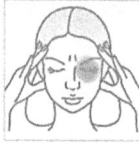

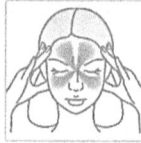

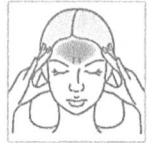

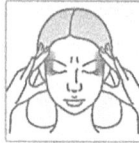

MIGRAINE CLUSTER SINUS TMJ TENSION

PAIN LEVEL

1	2	3	4	5	6	7	8	9	10

Not too bad. *Well, I'm not enjoying this.* *Make it stop!*

DETAILED DESCRIPTION

☐ Constant ☐ Squeezing ☐ Throbbing ☐ Pounding
☐ Dull aching ☐ Burning ☐ Sharp ☐ Debilitating

Other:____

ONSET

☐ Slow ☐ Average ☐ Rapid ☐ Sudden

WHERE DOES IT HURT, EXACTLY?

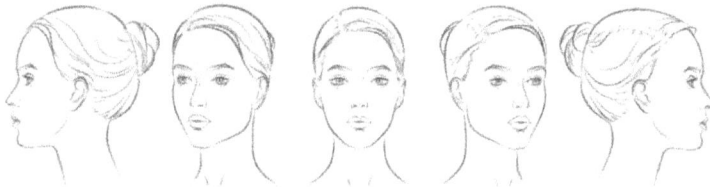

OTHER SYMPTOMS

☐ Lightheaded ☐ Dizziness ☐ Confusion
☐ Light sensitivity ☐ Sound sensitivity ☐ Auras
☐ Muscle stiffness ☐ Muscle burning ☐ Muscle aches

HOW ARE YOU FEELING OVERALL?

Mood	1	2	3	4	5	6	7	8	9	10
Energy levels	1	2	3	4	5	6	7	8	9	10
Mental clarity	1	2	3	4	5	6	7	8	9	10

Feeling sick?

☐ Nope!
☐ Yes...

☐ Nausea ☐ Diarrhea ☐ Vomiting ☐ Sore throat
☐ Congestion ☐ Coughing ☐ Chills ☐ Fever

Other symptoms: ________________________________

LAST NIGHT'S SLEEP

Hours of Sleep: ______________ Sleep Quality: ① ② ③ ④ ⑤

WEATHER

☐ Hot ☐ Mild ☐ Cold BM Pressure: ______

☐ Dry ☐ Humid ☐ Wet Allergen Levels: ______

☐ Sunny ☐ Cloudy

STRESS LEVELS

None	Low	Medium	High	Max	@$#%!

FOOD / DRINKS + NON-RELIEF MEDICATION / SUPPLEMENTS

item / meal	*time*	*meds / supplements*	*dose*	*time*

How many drinks?

water →	1	2	3	4	5	6	7	8	9	10
caffeine →	1	2	3	4	5	6	7	8	9	10
alcohol →	1	2	3	4	5	6	7	8	9	10

HORMONES

☐ Menstruating ☐ Menopause ☐ PMS ☐ N/A | other

COMPUTER USE / READING

☐ None ☐ Some ☐ A lot Total time: ______

☐ Sitting ☐ Standing ☐ Mixture Breaks every: ______

PHYSICAL ACTIVITY

☐ None ☐ Minimal ☐ Some ☐ Sweatin' ☐ I'm beat

DETAILS: ____

RELIEF MEASURES

☐ Medication ☐ Massage ☐ Sleep ☐ Exercise

☐ Water ☐ Cold/Ice ☐ Heat/Bath ☐ Other

DETAILS: ____

DID IT WORK? ☐ Nope ☐ A bit ☐ Mostly ☐ 100%

Notes

Entry #16

Date:________ M T W T F S S

START: | END: | DURATION:

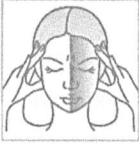

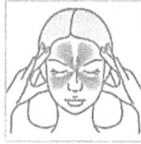

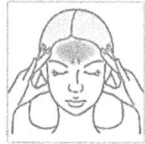

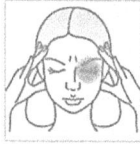

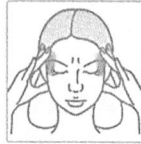

MIGRAINE CLUSTER SINUS TMJ TENSION

PAIN LEVEL

1	2	3	4	5	6	7	8	9	10

Not too bad. *Well, I'm not enjoying this.* *Make it stop!*

DETAILED DESCRIPTION

☐ Constant ☐ Squeezing ☐ Throbbing ☐ Pounding
☐ Dull aching ☐ Burning ☐ Sharp ☐ Debilitating

Other:______________________________

ONSET

☐ Slow ☐ Average ☐ Rapid ☐ Sudden

WHERE DOES IT HURT, EXACTLY?

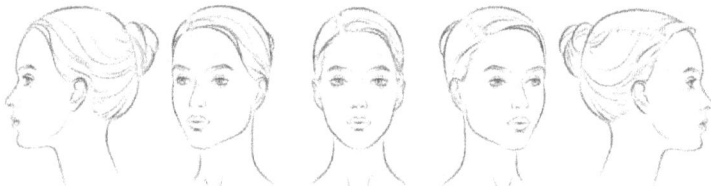

OTHER SYMPTOMS

☐ Lightheaded ☐ Dizziness ☐ Confusion
☐ Light sensitivity ☐ Sound sensitivity ☐ Auras
☐ Muscle stiffness ☐ Muscle burning ☐ Muscle aches

HOW ARE YOU FEELING OVERALL?

Mood	1	2	3	4	5	6	7	8	9	10
Energy levels	1	2	3	4	5	6	7	8	9	10
Mental clarity	1	2	3	4	5	6	7	8	9	10

Feeling sick?

☐ Nope!
☐ Yes...

☐ Nausea ☐ Diarrhea ☐ Vomiting ☐ Sore throat
☐ Congestion ☐ Coughing ☐ Chills ☐ Fever

Other symptoms:______________________________

LAST NIGHT'S SLEEP

Hours of Sleep: ____________ Sleep Quality: ① ② ③ ④ ⑤

WEATHER

☐ Hot ☐ Mild ☐ Cold BM Pressure: ______

☐ Dry ☐ Humid ☐ Wet Allergen Levels: ______

☐ Sunny ☐ Cloudy

STRESS LEVELS

None	Low	Medium	High	Max	@$#%!

FOOD / DRINKS + NON-RELIEF MEDICATION / SUPPLEMENTS

item / meal	*time*	*meds / supplements*	*dose*	*time*

How many drinks?

water	① ② ③ ④ ⑤ ⑥ ⑦ ⑧ ⑨ ⑩
caffeine	① ② ③ ④ ⑤ ⑥ ⑦ ⑧ ⑨ ⑩
alcohol	① ② ③ ④ ⑤ ⑥ ⑦ ⑧ ⑨ ⑩

HORMONES

☐ Menstruating ☐ Menopause ☐ PMS ☐ N/A | other

COMPUTER USE / READING

☐ None ☐ Some ☐ A lot Total time: ______

☐ Sitting ☐ Standing ☐ Mixture Breaks every: ______

PHYSICAL ACTIVITY

☐ None ☐ Minimal ☐ Some ☐ Sweatin' ☐ I'm beat

DETAILS: ______________________________

RELIEF MEASURES

☐ Medication ☐ Massage ☐ Sleep ☐ Exercise

☐ Water ☐ Cold/Ice ☐ Heat/Bath ☐ Other

DETAILS: ______________________________

DID IT WORK? ☐ Nope ☐ A bit ☐ Mostly ☐ 100%

Notes

Entry #17

Date:________ MTWTFSS

START:		END:		DURATION:	

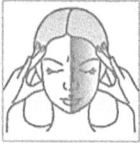

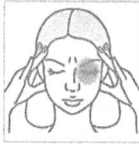

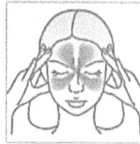

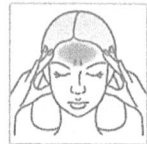

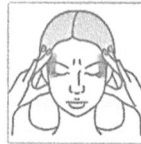

MIGRAINE CLUSTER SINUS TMJ TENSION

PAIN LEVEL

1	2	3	4	5	6	7	8	9	10

Not too bad. *Well, I'm not enjoying this.* *Make it stop!*

DETAILED DESCRIPTION

☐ Constant ☐ Squeezing ☐ Throbbing ☐ Pounding
☐ Dull aching ☐ Burning ☐ Sharp ☐ Debilitating

Other:______________________________

ONSET

☐ Slow ☐ Average ☐ Rapid ☐ Sudden

WHERE DOES IT HURT, EXACTLY?

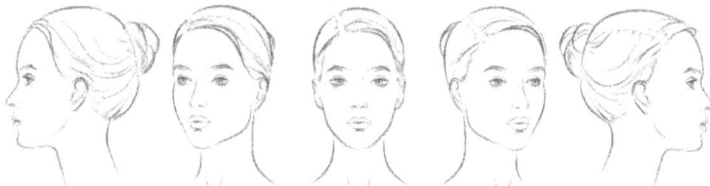

OTHER SYMPTOMS

☐ Lightheaded ☐ Dizziness ☐ Confusion
☐ Light sensitivity ☐ Sound sensitivity ☐ Auras
☐ Muscle stiffness ☐ Muscle burning ☐ Muscle aches

HOW ARE YOU FEELING OVERALL?

		Feeling sick?
Mood	① ② ③ ④ ⑤ ⑥ ⑦ ⑧ ⑨ ⑩	☐ Nope!
Energy levels	① ② ③ ④ ⑤ ⑥ ⑦ ⑧ ⑨ ⑩	☐ Yes...
Mental clarity	① ② ③ ④ ⑤ ⑥ ⑦ ⑧ ⑨ ⑩	

☐ Nausea ☐ Diarrhea ☐ Vomiting ☐ Sore throat
☐ Congestion ☐ Coughing ☐ Chills ☐ Fever

Other symptoms: ________________________

LAST NIGHT'S SLEEP

Hours of Sleep: ___________ Sleep Quality: ① ② ③ ④ ⑤

WEATHER

☐ Hot ☐ Mild ☐ Cold BM Pressure: ______

☐ Dry ☐ Humid ☐ Wet Allergen Levels: ______

☐ Sunny ☐ Cloudy

STRESS LEVELS

None	Low	Medium	High	Max	@$#%!

FOOD / DRINKS + NON-RELIEF MEDICATION / SUPPLEMENTS

item / meal	*time*	*meds / supplements*	*dose*	*time*

How many drinks?

water	① ② ③ ④ ⑤ ⑥ ⑦ ⑧ ⑨ ⑩
caffeine	① ② ③ ④ ⑤ ⑥ ⑦ ⑧ ⑨ ⑩
alcohol	① ② ③ ④ ⑤ ⑥ ⑦ ⑧ ⑨ ⑩

HORMONES

☐ Menstruating ☐ Menopause ☐ PMS ☐ N/A | other

COMPUTER USE / READING

☐ None ☐ Some ☐ A lot Total time:

☐ Sitting ☐ Standing ☐ Mixture Breaks every:

PHYSICAL ACTIVITY

☐ None ☐ Minimal ☐ Some ☐ Sweatin' ☐ I'm beat

DETAILS: ______________________________

RELIEF MEASURES

☐ Medication ☐ Massage ☐ Sleep ☐ Exercise

☐ Water ☐ Cold/Ice ☐ Heat/Bath ☐ Other

DETAILS: ______________________________

DID IT WORK? ☐ Nope ☐ A bit ☐ Mostly ☐ 100%

Notes

Entry #18

Date:________ M T W T F S S

START:		END:		DURATION:	

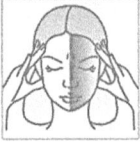

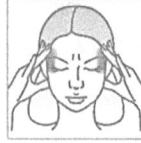

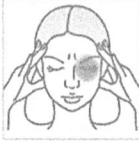

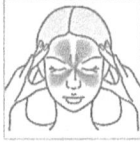

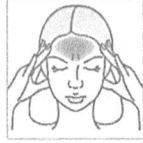

MIGRAINE CLUSTER SINUS TMJ TENSION

PAIN LEVEL

1	2	3	4	5	6	7	8	9	10

Not too bad. *Well, I'm not enjoying this.* *Make it stop!*

DETAILED DESCRIPTION

☐ Constant ☐ Squeezing ☐ Throbbing ☐ Pounding
☐ Dull aching ☐ Burning ☐ Sharp ☐ Debilitating

Other:________________________________

ONSET

☐ Slow ☐ Average ☐ Rapid ☐ Sudden

WHERE DOES IT HURT, EXACTLY?

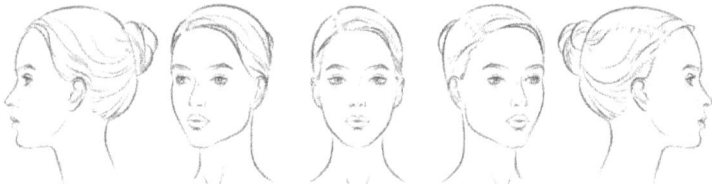

OTHER SYMPTOMS

☐ Lightheaded ☐ Dizziness ☐ Confusion
☐ Light sensitivity ☐ Sound sensitivity ☐ Auras
☐ Muscle stiffness ☐ Muscle burning ☐ Muscle aches

HOW ARE YOU FEELING OVERALL?

Mood	1	2	3	4	5	6	7	8	9	10
Energy levels	1	2	3	4	5	6	7	8	9	10
Mental clarity	1	2	3	4	5	6	7	8	9	10

Feeling sick?

☐ Nope!
☐ Yes...

☐ Nausea ☐ Diarrhea ☐ Vomiting ☐ Sore throat
☐ Congestion ☐ Coughing ☐ Chills ☐ Fever

Other symptoms: ________________________________

LAST NIGHT'S SLEEP

Hours of Sleep: ____________ Sleep Quality: ① ② ③ ④ ⑤

WEATHER

☐ Hot ☐ Mild ☐ Cold BM Pressure: ______

☐ Dry ☐ Humid ☐ Wet Allergen Levels: ______

☐ Sunny ☐ Cloudy

STRESS LEVELS

None	Low	Medium	High	Max	@$#%!

FOOD / DRINKS + NON-RELIEF MEDICATION / SUPPLEMENTS

item / meal	*time*	*meds / supplements*	*dose*	*time*

How many drinks?

water	1	2	3	4	5	6	7	8	9	10
caffeine	1	2	3	4	5	6	7	8	9	10
alcohol	1	2	3	4	5	6	7	8	9	10

HORMONES

☐ Menstruating ☐ Menopause ☐ PMS ☐ N/A | other

COMPUTER USE / READING

☐ None ☐ Some ☐ A lot Total time:

☐ Sitting ☐ Standing ☐ Mixture Breaks every:

PHYSICAL ACTIVITY

☐ None ☐ Minimal ☐ Some ☐ Sweatin' ☐ I'm beat

DETAILS: ______________________________

RELIEF MEASURES

☐ Medication ☐ Massage ☐ Sleep ☐ Exercise

☐ Water ☐ Cold/Ice ☐ Heat/Bath ☐ Other

DETAILS: ______________________________

DID IT WORK? ☐ Nope ☐ A bit ☐ Mostly ☐ 100%

Notes

Entry #19

Date:________ M T W T F S S

START:		END:		DURATION:	

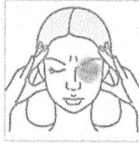

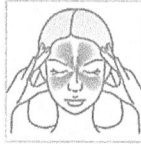

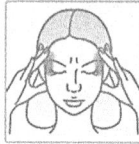

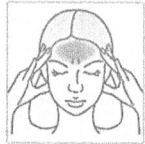

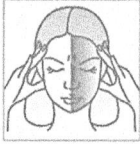

MIGRAINE CLUSTER SINUS TMJ TENSION

PAIN LEVEL

1	2	3	4	5	6	7	8	9	10

Not too bad. *Well, I'm not enjoying this.* *Make it stop!*

DETAILED DESCRIPTION

- ☐ Constant ☐ Squeezing ☐ Throbbing ☐ Pounding
- ☐ Dull aching ☐ Burning ☐ Sharp ☐ Debilitating

Other:________________________________

ONSET

☐ Slow ☐ Average ☐ Rapid ☐ Sudden

WHERE DOES IT HURT, EXACTLY?

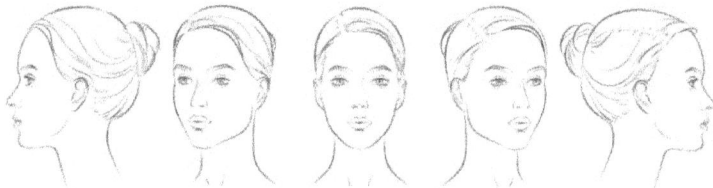

OTHER SYMPTOMS

- ☐ Lightheaded ☐ Dizziness ☐ Confusion
- ☐ Light sensitivity ☐ Sound sensitivity ☐ Auras
- ☐ Muscle stiffness ☐ Muscle burning ☐ Muscle aches

HOW ARE YOU FEELING OVERALL?

Mood	1	2	3	4	5	6	7	8	9	10
Energy levels	1	2	3	4	5	6	7	8	9	10
Mental clarity	1	2	3	4	5	6	7	8	9	10

Feeling sick?

☐ Nope!

☐ Yes...

- ☐ Nausea ☐ Diarrhea ☐ Vomiting ☐ Sore throat
- ☐ Congestion ☐ Coughing ☐ Chills ☐ Fever

Other symptoms: ________________________________

LAST NIGHT'S SLEEP

Hours of Sleep: ____________ Sleep Quality: ① ② ③ ④ ⑤

WEATHER

☐ Hot ☐ Mild ☐ Cold BM Pressure: ______

☐ Dry ☐ Humid ☐ Wet Allergen Levels: ______

☐ Sunny ☐ Cloudy

STRESS LEVELS

None	Low	Medium	High	Max	@$#%!

FOOD / DRINKS + NON-RELIEF MEDICATION / SUPPLEMENTS

item / meal	*time*	*meds / supplements*	*dose*	*time*

How many drinks?

water	→	① ② ③ ④ ⑤ ⑥ ⑦ ⑧ ⑨ ⑩
caffeine	→	① ② ③ ④ ⑤ ⑥ ⑦ ⑧ ⑨ ⑩
alcohol	→	① ② ③ ④ ⑤ ⑥ ⑦ ⑧ ⑨ ⑩

HORMONES

☐ Menstruating ☐ Menopause ☐ PMS ☐ N/A | other

COMPUTER USE / READING

☐ None ☐ Some ☐ A lot Total time:

☐ Sitting ☐ Standing ☐ Mixture Breaks every:

PHYSICAL ACTIVITY

☐ None ☐ Minimal ☐ Some ☐ Sweatin' ☐ I'm beat

DETAILS: ______________________________

RELIEF MEASURES

☐ Medication ☐ Massage ☐ Sleep ☐ Exercise

☐ Water ☐ Cold/Ice ☐ Heat/Bath ☐ Other

DETAILS: ______________________________

DID IT WORK? ☐ Nope ☐ A bit ☐ Mostly ☐ 100%

Notes

Entry #20

Date:________ M T W T F S S

START:		END:		DURATION:	

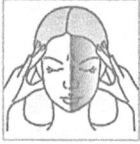

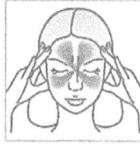

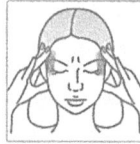

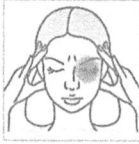

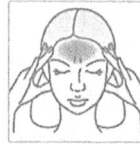

MIGRAINE CLUSTER SINUS TMJ TENSION

PAIN LEVEL

1	2	3	4	5	6	7	8	9	10

Not too bad. *Well, I'm not enjoying this.* *Make it stop!*

DETAILED DESCRIPTION

☐ Constant ☐ Squeezing ☐ Throbbing ☐ Pounding
☐ Dull aching ☐ Burning ☐ Sharp ☐ Debilitating

Other:____________________

ONSET

☐ Slow ☐ Average ☐ Rapid ☐ Sudden

WHERE DOES IT HURT, EXACTLY?

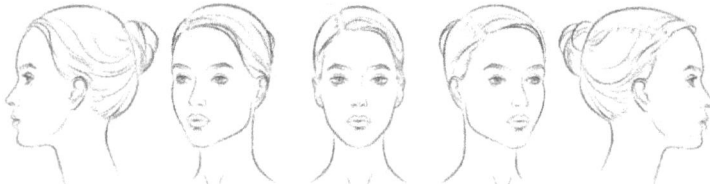

OTHER SYMPTOMS

☐ Lightheaded ☐ Dizziness ☐ Confusion
☐ Light sensitivity ☐ Sound sensitivity ☐ Auras
☐ Muscle stiffness ☐ Muscle burning ☐ Muscle aches

HOW ARE YOU FEELING OVERALL?

Mood	1	2	3	4	5	6	7	8	9	10
Energy levels	1	2	3	4	5	6	7	8	9	10
Mental clarity	1	2	3	4	5	6	7	8	9	10

Feeling sick?

☐ Nope!
☐ Yes...

☐ Nausea ☐ Diarrhea ☐ Vomiting ☐ Sore throat
☐ Congestion ☐ Coughing ☐ Chills ☐ Fever

Other symptoms: ____________________

LAST NIGHT'S SLEEP

Hours of Sleep: ______________ Sleep Quality: ① ② ③ ④ ⑤

WEATHER

☐ Hot ☐ Mild ☐ Cold BM Pressure: _______

☐ Dry ☐ Humid ☐ Wet Allergen Levels: _______

☐ Sunny ☐ Cloudy

STRESS LEVELS

None	Low	Medium	High	Max	@$#%!

FOOD / DRINKS + NON-RELIEF MEDICATION / SUPPLEMENTS

item / meal	*time*	*meds / supplements*	*dose*	*time*

How many drinks?

water	→	1	2	3	4	5	6	7	8	9	10
caffeine	→	1	2	3	4	5	6	7	8	9	10
alcohol	→	1	2	3	4	5	6	7	8	9	10

HORMONES

☐ Menstruating ☐ Menopause ☐ PMS ☐ N/A | other

COMPUTER USE / READING

☐ None ☐ Some ☐ A lot Total time: ☐

☐ Sitting ☐ Standing ☐ Mixture Breaks every: ☐

PHYSICAL ACTIVITY

☐ None ☐ Minimal ☐ Some ☐ Sweatin' ☐ I'm beat

DETAILS: ______________________________

RELIEF MEASURES

☐ Medication ☐ Massage ☐ Sleep ☐ Exercise

☐ Water ☐ Cold/Ice ☐ Heat/Bath ☐ Other

DETAILS: ______________________________

DID IT WORK? ☐ Nope ☐ A bit ☐ Mostly ☐ 100%

Notes

Entry #21

Date:________ M T W T F S S

START:		END:		DURATION:	

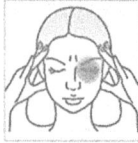

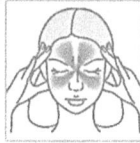

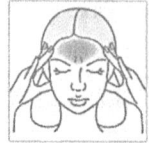

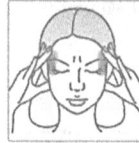

MIGRAINE CLUSTER SINUS TMJ TENSION

PAIN LEVEL

1	2	3	4	5	6	7	8	9	10

Not too bad. *Well, I'm not enjoying this.* *Make it stop!*

DETAILED DESCRIPTION

☐ Constant ☐ Squeezing ☐ Throbbing ☐ Pounding
☐ Dull aching ☐ Burning ☐ Sharp ☐ Debilitating

Other:________________________________

ONSET

☐ Slow ☐ Average ☐ Rapid ☐ Sudden

WHERE DOES IT HURT, EXACTLY?

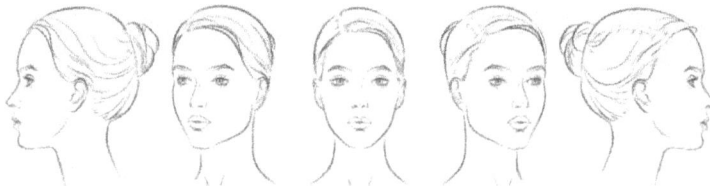

OTHER SYMPTOMS

☐ Lightheaded ☐ Dizziness ☐ Confusion
☐ Light sensitivity ☐ Sound sensitivity ☐ Auras
☐ Muscle stiffness ☐ Muscle burning ☐ Muscle aches

HOW ARE YOU FEELING OVERALL?

		Feeling sick?
Mood	① ② ③ ④ ⑤ ⑥ ⑦ ⑧ ⑨ ⑩	☐ Nope!
Energy levels	① ② ③ ④ ⑤ ⑥ ⑦ ⑧ ⑨ ⑩	☐ Yes…
Mental clarity	① ② ③ ④ ⑤ ⑥ ⑦ ⑧ ⑨ ⑩	

☐ Nausea ☐ Diarrhea ☐ Vomiting ☐ Sore throat
☐ Congestion ☐ Coughing ☐ Chills ☐ Fever

Other symptoms: ________________________________

LAST NIGHT'S SLEEP

Hours of Sleep: ____________ Sleep Quality: ① ② ③ ④ ⑤

WEATHER

☐ Hot ☐ Mild ☐ Cold BM Pressure: ______

☐ Dry ☐ Humid ☐ Wet Allergen Levels: ______

☐ Sunny ☐ Cloudy

STRESS LEVELS

None	Low	Medium	High	Max	@$#%!

FOOD / DRINKS + NON-RELIEF MEDICATION / SUPPLEMENTS

item / meal	*time*	*meds / supplements*	*dose*	*time*

How many drinks?

water →	① ② ③ ④ ⑤ ⑥ ⑦ ⑧ ⑨ ⑩
caffeine →	① ② ③ ④ ⑤ ⑥ ⑦ ⑧ ⑨ ⑩
alcohol →	① ② ③ ④ ⑤ ⑥ ⑦ ⑧ ⑨ ⑩

HORMONES

☐ Menstruating ☐ Menopause ☐ PMS ☐ N/A | other

COMPUTER USE / READING

☐ None ☐ Some ☐ A lot Total time: ______

☐ Sitting ☐ Standing ☐ Mixture Breaks every: ______

PHYSICAL ACTIVITY

☐ None ☐ Minimal ☐ Some ☐ Sweatin' ☐ I'm beat

DETAILS: ______________________________

RELIEF MEASURES

☐ Medication ☐ Massage ☐ Sleep ☐ Exercise

☐ Water ☐ Cold/Ice ☐ Heat/Bath ☐ Other

DETAILS: ______________________________

DID IT WORK? ☐ Nope ☐ A bit ☐ Mostly ☐ 100%

Notes

Entry #22

Date:________ M T W T F S S

START:		END:		DURATION:	

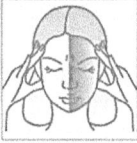

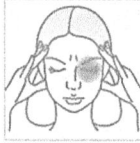

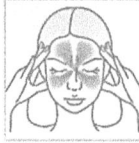

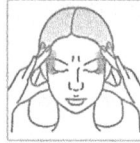

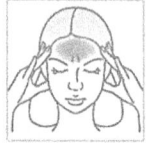

MIGRAINE CLUSTER SINUS TMJ TENSION

PAIN LEVEL

1	2	3	4	5	6	7	8	9	10

Not too bad. *Well, I'm not enjoying this.* *Make it stop!*

DETAILED DESCRIPTION

☐ Constant ☐ Squeezing ☐ Throbbing ☐ Pounding
☐ Dull aching ☐ Burning ☐ Sharp ☐ Debilitating

Other:____________________

ONSET

☐ Slow ☐ Average ☐ Rapid ☐ Sudden

WHERE DOES IT HURT, EXACTLY?

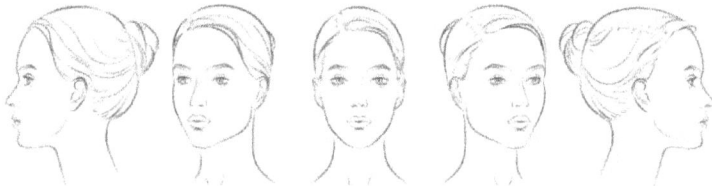

OTHER SYMPTOMS

☐ Lightheaded ☐ Dizziness ☐ Confusion
☐ Light sensitivity ☐ Sound sensitivity ☐ Auras
☐ Muscle stiffness ☐ Muscle burning ☐ Muscle aches

HOW ARE YOU FEELING OVERALL?

Mood	1	2	3	4	5	6	7	8	9	10
Energy levels	1	2	3	4	5	6	7	8	9	10
Mental clarity	1	2	3	4	5	6	7	8	9	10

Feeling sick?

☐ Nope!
☐ Yes...

☐ Nausea ☐ Diarrhea ☐ Vomiting ☐ Sore throat
☐ Congestion ☐ Coughing ☐ Chills ☐ Fever

Other symptoms: ____________________

LAST NIGHT'S SLEEP

Hours of Sleep: ____________ Sleep Quality: ① ② ③ ④ ⑤

WEATHER

☐ Hot ☐ Mild ☐ Cold BM Pressure: ______

☐ Dry ☐ Humid ☐ Wet Allergen Levels: ______

☐ Sunny ☐ Cloudy

STRESS LEVELS

None	Low	Medium	High	Max	@$#%!

FOOD / DRINKS + NON-RELIEF MEDICATION / SUPPLEMENTS

item / meal	*time*	*meds / supplements*	*dose*	*time*

How many drinks?

water	① ② ③ ④ ⑤ ⑥ ⑦ ⑧ ⑨ ⑩
caffeine	① ② ③ ④ ⑤ ⑥ ⑦ ⑧ ⑨ ⑩
alcohol	① ② ③ ④ ⑤ ⑥ ⑦ ⑧ ⑨ ⑩

HORMONES

☐ Menstruating ☐ Menopause ☐ PMS ☐ N/A | other

COMPUTER USE / READING

☐ None ☐ Some ☐ A lot Total time:

☐ Sitting ☐ Standing ☐ Mixture Breaks every:

PHYSICAL ACTIVITY

☐ None ☐ Minimal ☐ Some ☐ Sweatin' ☐ I'm beat

DETAILS: ____________________

RELIEF MEASURES

☐ Medication ☐ Massage ☐ Sleep ☐ Exercise

☐ Water ☐ Cold/Ice ☐ Heat/Bath ☐ Other

DETAILS: ____________________

DID IT WORK? ☐ Nope ☐ A bit ☐ Mostly ☐ 100%

Notes

Entry #23

Date:________ M T W T F S S

START:		END:		DURATION:	

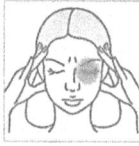

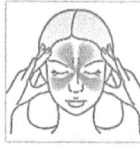

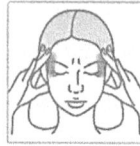

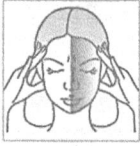

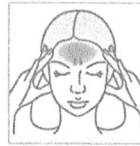

MIGRAINE CLUSTER SINUS TMJ TENSION

PAIN LEVEL

1	2	3	4	5	6	7	8	9	10

Not too bad. *Well, I'm not enjoying this.* *Make it stop!*

DETAILED DESCRIPTION

☐ Constant ☐ Squeezing ☐ Throbbing ☐ Pounding
☐ Dull aching ☐ Burning ☐ Sharp ☐ Debilitating

Other:________________________________

ONSET

☐ Slow ☐ Average ☐ Rapid ☐ Sudden

WHERE DOES IT HURT, EXACTLY?

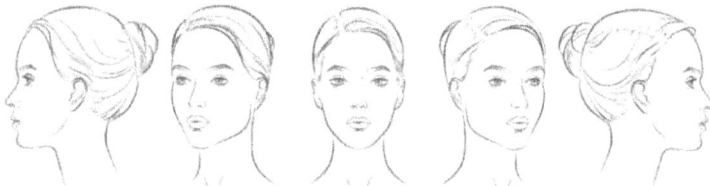

OTHER SYMPTOMS

☐ Lightheaded ☐ Dizziness ☐ Confusion
☐ Light sensitivity ☐ Sound sensitivity ☐ Auras
☐ Muscle stiffness ☐ Muscle burning ☐ Muscle aches

HOW ARE YOU FEELING OVERALL?

Mood	① ② ③ ④ ⑤ ⑥ ⑦ ⑧ ⑨ ⑩	
Energy levels	① ② ③ ④ ⑤ ⑥ ⑦ ⑧ ⑨ ⑩	
Mental clarity	① ② ③ ④ ⑤ ⑥ ⑦ ⑧ ⑨ ⑩	

Feeling sick?

☐ Nope!
☐ Yes...

☐ Nausea ☐ Diarrhea ☐ Vomiting ☐ Sore throat
☐ Congestion ☐ Coughing ☐ Chills ☐ Fever

Other symptoms: ________________________________

LAST NIGHT'S SLEEP

Hours of Sleep: ____________ Sleep Quality: ① ② ③ ④ ⑤

WEATHER

☐ Hot ☐ Mild ☐ Cold BM Pressure: ______

☐ Dry ☐ Humid ☐ Wet Allergen Levels: ______

☐ Sunny ☐ Cloudy

STRESS LEVELS

None	Low	Medium	High	Max	@$#%!

FOOD / DRINKS + NON-RELIEF MEDICATION / SUPPLEMENTS

item / meal	*time*	*meds / supplements*	*dose*	*time*

How many drinks?

water	⇨	① ② ③ ④ ⑤ ⑥ ⑦ ⑧ ⑨ ⑩
caffeine	⇨	① ② ③ ④ ⑤ ⑥ ⑦ ⑧ ⑨ ⑩
alcohol	⇨	① ② ③ ④ ⑤ ⑥ ⑦ ⑧ ⑨ ⑩

HORMONES

☐ Menstruating ☐ Menopause ☐ PMS ☐ N/A | other

COMPUTER USE / READING

☐ None ☐ Some ☐ A lot Total time: [ ]

☐ Sitting ☐ Standing ☐ Mixture Breaks every: [ ]

PHYSICAL ACTIVITY

☐ None ☐ Minimal ☐ Some ☐ Sweatin' ☐ I'm beat

DETAILS: ________________________________

RELIEF MEASURES

☐ Medication ☐ Massage ☐ Sleep ☐ Exercise

☐ Water ☐ Cold/Ice ☐ Heat/Bath ☐ Other

DETAILS: ________________________________

DID IT WORK? ☐ Nope ☐ A bit ☐ Mostly ☐ 100%

Notes

Entry #24

Date:________ M T W T F S S

START:		END:		DURATION:	

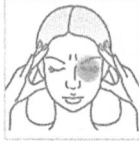

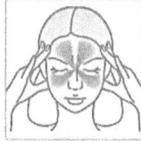

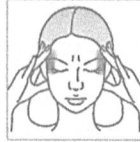

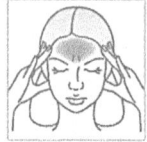

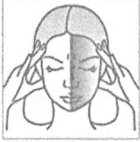

MIGRAINE CLUSTER SINUS TMJ TENSION

PAIN LEVEL

1	2	3	4	5	6	7	8	9	10

Not too bad. *Well, I'm not enjoying this.* *Make it stop!*

DETAILED DESCRIPTION

☐ Constant ☐ Squeezing ☐ Throbbing ☐ Pounding
☐ Dull aching ☐ Burning ☐ Sharp ☐ Debilitating

Other:______________________________

ONSET

☐ Slow ☐ Average ☐ Rapid ☐ Sudden

WHERE DOES IT HURT, EXACTLY?

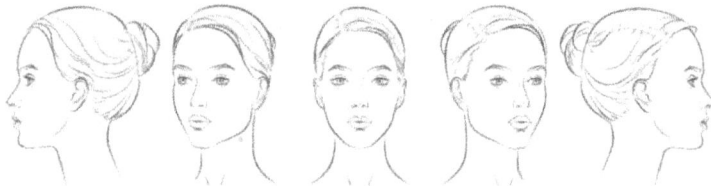

OTHER SYMPTOMS

☐ Lightheaded ☐ Dizziness ☐ Confusion
☐ Light sensitivity ☐ Sound sensitivity ☐ Auras
☐ Muscle stiffness ☐ Muscle burning ☐ Muscle aches

HOW ARE YOU FEELING OVERALL?

Mood	1	2	3	4	5	6	7	8	9	10
Energy levels	1	2	3	4	5	6	7	8	9	10
Mental clarity	1	2	3	4	5	6	7	8	9	10

Feeling sick?

☐ Nope!
☐ Yes...

☐ Nausea ☐ Diarrhea ☐ Vomiting ☐ Sore throat
☐ Congestion ☐ Coughing ☐ Chills ☐ Fever

Other symptoms: ______________________________

LAST NIGHT'S SLEEP

Hours of Sleep: ______________ Sleep Quality: ① ② ③ ④ ⑤

WEATHER

☐ Hot ☐ Mild ☐ Cold BM Pressure: _______

☐ Dry ☐ Humid ☐ Wet Allergen Levels: _______

☐ Sunny ☐ Cloudy

STRESS LEVELS

None	Low	Medium	High	Max	@$#%!

FOOD / DRINKS + NON-RELIEF MEDICATION / SUPPLEMENTS

item / meal	*time*	*meds / supplements*	*dose*	*time*

How many drinks?

water →	① ② ③ ④ ⑤ ⑥ ⑦ ⑧ ⑨ ⑩
caffeine →	① ② ③ ④ ⑤ ⑥ ⑦ ⑧ ⑨ ⑩
alcohol →	① ② ③ ④ ⑤ ⑥ ⑦ ⑧ ⑨ ⑩

HORMONES

☐ Menstruating ☐ Menopause ☐ PMS ☐ N/A | other

COMPUTER USE / READING

☐ None ☐ Some ☐ A lot Total time: ☐

☐ Sitting ☐ Standing ☐ Mixture Breaks every: ☐

PHYSICAL ACTIVITY

☐ None ☐ Minimal ☐ Some ☐ Sweatin' ☐ I'm beat

DETAILS: ____

RELIEF MEASURES

☐ Medication ☐ Massage ☐ Sleep ☐ Exercise

☐ Water ☐ Cold/Ice ☐ Heat/Bath ☐ Other

DETAILS: ____

DID IT WORK? ☐ Nope ☐ A bit ☐ Mostly ☐ 100%

Notes

Entry #25

Date:________ M T W T F S S

START: | END: | DURATION:

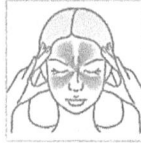

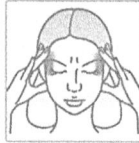

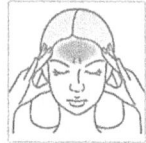

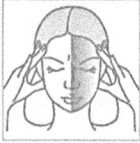

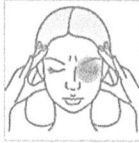

MIGRAINE CLUSTER SINUS TMJ TENSION

PAIN LEVEL

1	2	3	4	5	6	7	8	9	10

Not too bad. *Well, I'm not enjoying this.* *Make it stop!*

DETAILED DESCRIPTION

☐ Constant ☐ Squeezing ☐ Throbbing ☐ Pounding
☐ Dull aching ☐ Burning ☐ Sharp ☐ Debilitating

Other:________________________________

ONSET

☐ Slow ☐ Average ☐ Rapid ☐ Sudden

WHERE DOES IT HURT, EXACTLY?

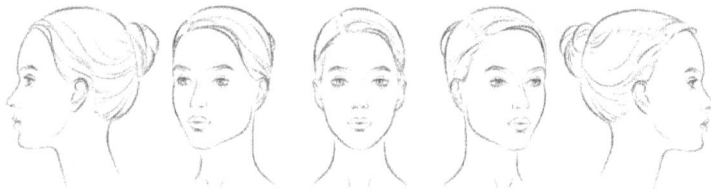

OTHER SYMPTOMS

☐ Lightheaded ☐ Dizziness ☐ Confusion
☐ Light sensitivity ☐ Sound sensitivity ☐ Auras
☐ Muscle stiffness ☐ Muscle burning ☐ Muscle aches

HOW ARE YOU FEELING OVERALL?

Mood	① ② ③ ④ ⑤ ⑥ ⑦ ⑧ ⑨ ⑩
Energy levels	① ② ③ ④ ⑤ ⑥ ⑦ ⑧ ⑨ ⑩
Mental clarity	① ② ③ ④ ⑤ ⑥ ⑦ ⑧ ⑨ ⑩

Feeling sick?

☐ Nope!
☐ Yes...

☐ Nausea ☐ Diarrhea ☐ Vomiting ☐ Sore throat
☐ Congestion ☐ Coughing ☐ Chills ☐ Fever

Other symptoms: ________________________________

LAST NIGHT'S SLEEP

Hours of Sleep: ________ Sleep Quality: ① ② ③ ④ ⑤

WEATHER

☐ Hot ☐ Mild ☐ Cold BM Pressure: ______

☐ Dry ☐ Humid ☐ Wet Allergen Levels: ______

☐ Sunny ☐ Cloudy

STRESS LEVELS

None	Low	Medium	High	Max	@$#%!

FOOD / DRINKS + NON-RELIEF MEDICATION / SUPPLEMENTS

item / meal	*time*	*meds / supplements*	*dose*	*time*

How many drinks?

water	① ② ③ ④ ⑤ ⑥ ⑦ ⑧ ⑨ ⑩
caffeine	① ② ③ ④ ⑤ ⑥ ⑦ ⑧ ⑨ ⑩
alcohol	① ② ③ ④ ⑤ ⑥ ⑦ ⑧ ⑨ ⑩

HORMONES

☐ Menstruating ☐ Menopause ☐ PMS ☐ N/A | other

COMPUTER USE / READING

☐ None ☐ Some ☐ A lot Total time:

☐ Sitting ☐ Standing ☐ Mixture Breaks every:

PHYSICAL ACTIVITY

☐ None ☐ Minimal ☐ Some ☐ Sweatin' ☐ I'm beat

DETAILS: ________

RELIEF MEASURES

☐ Medication ☐ Massage ☐ Sleep ☐ Exercise

☐ Water ☐ Cold/Ice ☐ Heat/Bath ☐ Other

DETAILS: ________

DID IT WORK? ☐ Nope ☐ A bit ☐ Mostly ☐ 100%

Notes

Entry #26

Date:________ M T W T F S S

START:		END:		DURATION:	

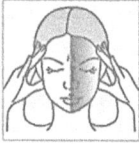

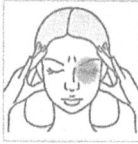

MIGRAINE CLUSTER SINUS TMJ TENSION

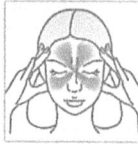

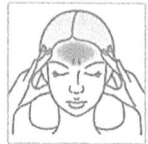

PAIN LEVEL

1	2	3	4	5	6	7	8	9	10

Not too bad. *Well, I'm not enjoying this.* *Make it stop!*

DETAILED DESCRIPTION

☐ Constant ☐ Squeezing ☐ Throbbing ☐ Pounding
☐ Dull aching ☐ Burning ☐ Sharp ☐ Debilitating

Other:________________________________

ONSET

☐ Slow ☐ Average ☐ Rapid ☐ Sudden

WHERE DOES IT HURT, EXACTLY?

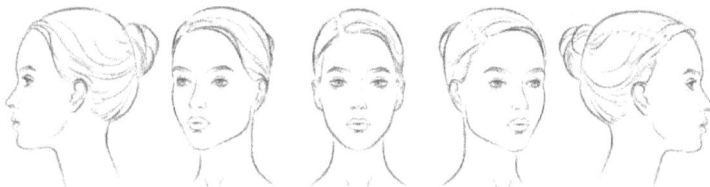

OTHER SYMPTOMS

☐ Lightheaded ☐ Dizziness ☐ Confusion
☐ Light sensitivity ☐ Sound sensitivity ☐ Auras
☐ Muscle stiffness ☐ Muscle burning ☐ Muscle aches

HOW ARE YOU FEELING OVERALL?

		Feeling sick?
Mood	① ② ③ ④ ⑤ ⑥ ⑦ ⑧ ⑨ ⑩	☐ Nope!
Energy levels	① ② ③ ④ ⑤ ⑥ ⑦ ⑧ ⑨ ⑩	☐ Yes...
Mental clarity	① ② ③ ④ ⑤ ⑥ ⑦ ⑧ ⑨ ⑩	

☐ Nausea ☐ Diarrhea ☐ Vomiting ☐ Sore throat
☐ Congestion ☐ Coughing ☐ Chills ☐ Fever

Other symptoms: ________________________

LAST NIGHT'S SLEEP

Hours of Sleep: ____________ Sleep Quality: ① ② ③ ④ ⑤

WEATHER

☐ Hot ☐ Mild ☐ Cold BM Pressure: ______
☐ Dry ☐ Humid ☐ Wet Allergen Levels: ______
☐ Sunny ☐ Cloudy

STRESS LEVELS

None	Low	Medium	High	Max	@$#%!

FOOD / DRINKS + NON-RELIEF MEDICATION / SUPPLEMENTS

item / meal	*time*	*meds / supplements*	*dose*	*time*

How many drinks?

water	① ② ③ ④ ⑤ ⑥ ⑦ ⑧ ⑨ ⑩
caffeine	① ② ③ ④ ⑤ ⑥ ⑦ ⑧ ⑨ ⑩
alcohol	① ② ③ ④ ⑤ ⑥ ⑦ ⑧ ⑨ ⑩

HORMONES

☐ Menstruating ☐ Menopause ☐ PMS ☐ N/A | other

COMPUTER USE / READING

☐ None ☐ Some ☐ A lot Total time:
☐ Sitting ☐ Standing ☐ Mixture Breaks every:

PHYSICAL ACTIVITY

☐ None ☐ Minimal ☐ Some ☐ Sweatin' ☐ I'm beat

DETAILS: ____________________

RELIEF MEASURES

☐ Medication ☐ Massage ☐ Sleep ☐ Exercise
☐ Water ☐ Cold/Ice ☐ Heat/Bath ☐ Other

DETAILS: ____________________

DID IT WORK? ☐ Nope ☐ A bit ☐ Mostly ☐ 100%

Notes

Entry #27

Date:________ **M T W T F S S**

START:		END:		DURATION:	

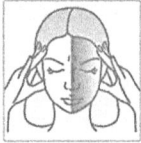

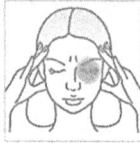

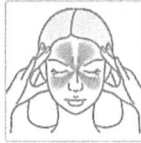

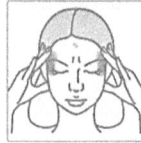

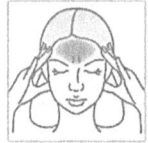

MIGRAINE CLUSTER SINUS TMJ TENSION

PAIN LEVEL

1	2	3	4	5	6	7	8	9	10

Not too bad. *Well, I'm not enjoying this.* *Make it stop!*

DETAILED DESCRIPTION

☐ Constant ☐ Squeezing ☐ Throbbing ☐ Pounding
☐ Dull aching ☐ Burning ☐ Sharp ☐ Debilitating

Other:______________________

ONSET

☐ Slow ☐ Average ☐ Rapid ☐ Sudden

WHERE DOES IT HURT, EXACTLY?

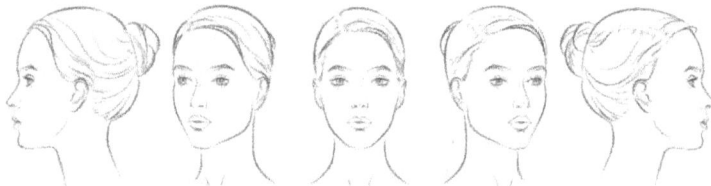

OTHER SYMPTOMS

☐ Lightheaded ☐ Dizziness ☐ Confusion
☐ Light sensitivity ☐ Sound sensitivity ☐ Auras
☐ Muscle stiffness ☐ Muscle burning ☐ Muscle aches

HOW ARE YOU FEELING OVERALL?

		Feeling sick?
Mood	① ② ③ ④ ⑤ ⑥ ⑦ ⑧ ⑨ ⑩	☐ Nope!
Energy levels	① ② ③ ④ ⑤ ⑥ ⑦ ⑧ ⑨ ⑩	☐ Yes...
Mental clarity	① ② ③ ④ ⑤ ⑥ ⑦ ⑧ ⑨ ⑩	

☐ Nausea ☐ Diarrhea ☐ Vomiting ☐ Sore throat
☐ Congestion ☐ Coughing ☐ Chills ☐ Fever

Other symptoms: ______________________

LAST NIGHT'S SLEEP

Hours of Sleep: ____________ Sleep Quality: ① ② ③ ④ ⑤

WEATHER

☐ Hot ☐ Mild ☐ Cold BM Pressure: ______

☐ Dry ☐ Humid ☐ Wet Allergen Levels: ______

☐ Sunny ☐ Cloudy

STRESS LEVELS

None	Low	Medium	High	Max	@$#%!

FOOD / DRINKS + NON-RELIEF MEDICATION / SUPPLEMENTS

item / meal	*time*	*meds / supplements*	*dose*	*time*
		How many drinks?		

water → ① ② ③ ④ ⑤ ⑥ ⑦ ⑧ ⑨ ⑩

caffeine → ① ② ③ ④ ⑤ ⑥ ⑦ ⑧ ⑨ ⑩

alcohol → ① ② ③ ④ ⑤ ⑥ ⑦ ⑧ ⑨ ⑩

HORMONES

☐ Menstruating ☐ Menopause ☐ PMS ☐ N/A | other

COMPUTER USE / READING

☐ None ☐ Some ☐ A lot Total time:

☐ Sitting ☐ Standing ☐ Mixture Breaks every:

PHYSICAL ACTIVITY

☐ None ☐ Minimal ☐ Some ☐ Sweatin' ☐ I'm beat

DETAILS: ____________________

RELIEF MEASURES

☐ Medication ☐ Massage ☐ Sleep ☐ Exercise

☐ Water ☐ Cold/Ice ☐ Heat/Bath ☐ Other

DETAILS: ____________________

DID IT WORK? ☐ Nope ☐ A bit ☐ Mostly ☐ 100%

Notes

Entry #28

Date:________ M T W T F S S

START: END: DURATION:

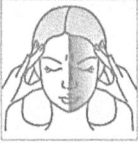

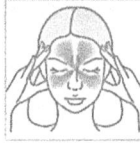

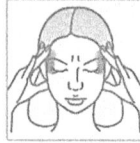

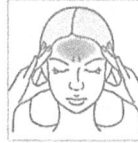

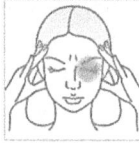

MIGRAINE CLUSTER SINUS TMJ TENSION

PAIN LEVEL

1	2	3	4	5	6	7	8	9	10

Not too bad. *Well, I'm not enjoying this.* *Make it stop!*

DETAILED DESCRIPTION

☐ Constant ☐ Squeezing ☐ Throbbing ☐ Pounding
☐ Dull aching ☐ Burning ☐ Sharp ☐ Debilitating

Other:________________________________

ONSET

☐ Slow ☐ Average ☐ Rapid ☐ Sudden

WHERE DOES IT HURT, EXACTLY?

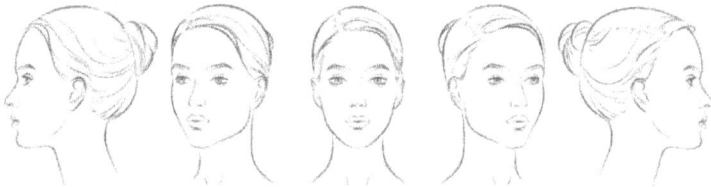

OTHER SYMPTOMS

☐ Lightheaded ☐ Dizziness ☐ Confusion
☐ Light sensitivity ☐ Sound sensitivity ☐ Auras
☐ Muscle stiffness ☐ Muscle burning ☐ Muscle aches

HOW ARE YOU FEELING OVERALL?

		Feeling sick?
Mood	① ② ③ ④ ⑤ ⑥ ⑦ ⑧ ⑨ ⑩	☐ Nope!
Energy levels	① ② ③ ④ ⑤ ⑥ ⑦ ⑧ ⑨ ⑩	☐ Yes...
Mental clarity	① ② ③ ④ ⑤ ⑥ ⑦ ⑧ ⑨ ⑩	

☐ Nausea ☐ Diarrhea ☐ Vomiting ☐ Sore throat
☐ Congestion ☐ Coughing ☐ Chills ☐ Fever

Other symptoms:________________________________

LAST NIGHT'S SLEEP

Hours of Sleep: ____________ Sleep Quality: ① ② ③ ④ ⑤

WEATHER

☐ Hot ☐ Mild ☐ Cold BM Pressure: ______

☐ Dry ☐ Humid ☐ Wet Allergen Levels: ______

☐ Sunny ☐ Cloudy

STRESS LEVELS

None	Low	Medium	High	Max	@$#%!

FOOD / DRINKS + NON-RELIEF MEDICATION / SUPPLEMENTS

item / meal	*time*	*meds / supplements*	*dose*	*time*

How many drinks?

water	⇒	① ② ③ ④ ⑤ ⑥ ⑦ ⑧ ⑨ ⑩
caffeine	⇒	① ② ③ ④ ⑤ ⑥ ⑦ ⑧ ⑨ ⑩
alcohol	⇒	① ② ③ ④ ⑤ ⑥ ⑦ ⑧ ⑨ ⑩

HORMONES

☐ Menstruating ☐ Menopause ☐ PMS ☐ N/A | other

COMPUTER USE / READING

☐ None ☐ Some ☐ A lot Total time: ______

☐ Sitting ☐ Standing ☐ Mixture Breaks every: ______

PHYSICAL ACTIVITY

☐ None ☐ Minimal ☐ Some ☐ Sweatin' ☐ I'm beat

DETAILS: ________________________________

RELIEF MEASURES

☐ Medication ☐ Massage ☐ Sleep ☐ Exercise

☐ Water ☐ Cold/Ice ☐ Heat/Bath ☐ Other

DETAILS: ________________________________

DID IT WORK? ☐ Nope ☐ A bit ☐ Mostly ☐ 100%

Notes

Entry #29

Date:________ M T W T F S S

START:		END:		DURATION:	

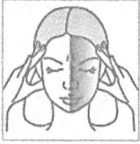

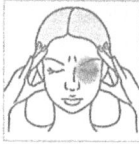

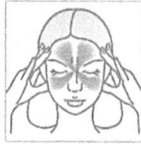

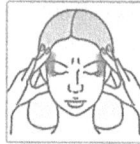

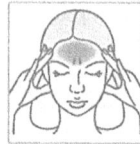

MIGRAINE CLUSTER SINUS TMJ TENSION

PAIN LEVEL

1	2	3	4	5	6	7	8	9	10

Not too bad. *Well, I'm not enjoying this.* *Make it stop!*

DETAILED DESCRIPTION

☐ Constant ☐ Squeezing ☐ Throbbing ☐ Pounding
☐ Dull aching ☐ Burning ☐ Sharp ☐ Debilitating

Other:____________________

ONSET

☐ Slow ☐ Average ☐ Rapid ☐ Sudden

WHERE DOES IT HURT, EXACTLY?

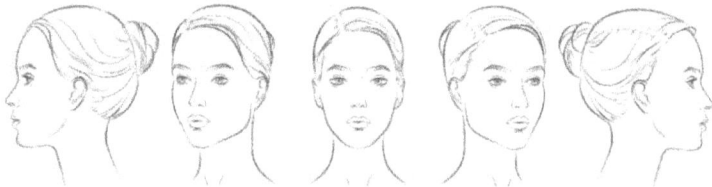

OTHER SYMPTOMS

☐ Lightheaded ☐ Dizziness ☐ Confusion
☐ Light sensitivity ☐ Sound sensitivity ☐ Auras
☐ Muscle stiffness ☐ Muscle burning ☐ Muscle aches

HOW ARE YOU FEELING OVERALL?

Mood	1	2	3	4	5	6	7	8	9	10
Energy levels	1	2	3	4	5	6	7	8	9	10
Mental clarity	1	2	3	4	5	6	7	8	9	10

Feeling sick?

☐ Nope!
☐ Yes...

☐ Nausea ☐ Diarrhea ☐ Vomiting ☐ Sore throat
☐ Congestion ☐ Coughing ☐ Chills ☐ Fever

Other symptoms: ____________________

LAST NIGHT'S SLEEP

Hours of Sleep: ______________ Sleep Quality: (1) (2) (3) (4) (5)

WEATHER

☐ Hot ☐ Mild ☐ Cold BM Pressure: _______

☐ Dry ☐ Humid ☐ Wet Allergen Levels: _______

☐ Sunny ☐ Cloudy

STRESS LEVELS

None	Low	Medium	High	Max	@$#%!

FOOD / DRINKS + NON-RELIEF MEDICATION / SUPPLEMENTS

item / meal	*time*	*meds / supplements*	*dose*	*time*

How many drinks?

water	(1) (2) (3) (4) (5) (6) (7) (8) (9) (10)
caffeine	(1) (2) (3) (4) (5) (6) (7) (8) (9) (10)
alcohol	(1) (2) (3) (4) (5) (6) (7) (8) (9) (10)

HORMONES

☐ Menstruating ☐ Menopause ☐ PMS ☐ N/A | other

COMPUTER USE / READING

☐ None ☐ Some ☐ A lot Total time: ☐

☐ Sitting ☐ Standing ☐ Mixture Breaks every: ☐

PHYSICAL ACTIVITY

☐ None ☐ Minimal ☐ Some ☐ Sweatin' ☐ I'm beat

DETAILS: ______________________________________

RELIEF MEASURES

☐ Medication ☐ Massage ☐ Sleep ☐ Exercise

☐ Water ☐ Cold/Ice ☐ Heat/Bath ☐ Other

DETAILS: ______________________________________

DID IT WORK? ☐ Nope ☐ A bit ☐ Mostly ☐ 100%

Notes

Entry #30

Date:________ M T W T F S S

START:		END:		DURATION:	

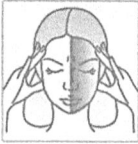

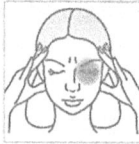

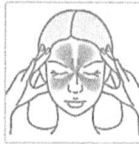

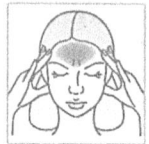

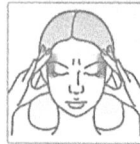

MIGRAINE CLUSTER SINUS TMJ TENSION

PAIN LEVEL

1	2	3	4	5	6	7	8	9	10

Not too bad. *Well, I'm not enjoying this.* *Make it stop!*

DETAILED DESCRIPTION

☐ Constant ☐ Squeezing ☐ Throbbing ☐ Pounding
☐ Dull aching ☐ Burning ☐ Sharp ☐ Debilitating

Other:____

ONSET

☐ Slow ☐ Average ☐ Rapid ☐ Sudden

WHERE DOES IT HURT, EXACTLY?

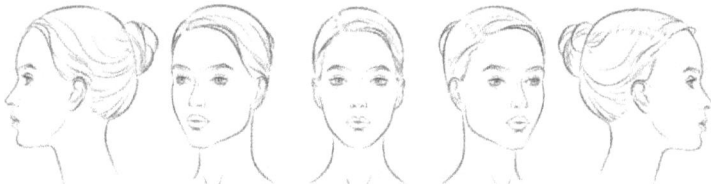

OTHER SYMPTOMS

☐ Lightheaded ☐ Dizziness ☐ Confusion
☐ Light sensitivity ☐ Sound sensitivity ☐ Auras
☐ Muscle stiffness ☐ Muscle burning ☐ Muscle aches

HOW ARE YOU FEELING OVERALL?

Mood	1	2	3	4	5	6	7	8	9	10
Energy levels	1	2	3	4	5	6	7	8	9	10
Mental clarity	1	2	3	4	5	6	7	8	9	10

Feeling sick?

☐ Nope!
☐ Yes...

☐ Nausea ☐ Diarrhea ☐ Vomiting ☐ Sore throat
☐ Congestion ☐ Coughing ☐ Chills ☐ Fever

Other symptoms: ______________________________

LAST NIGHT'S SLEEP

Hours of Sleep: ______________ Sleep Quality: ① ② ③ ④ ⑤

WEATHER

☐ Hot ☐ Mild ☐ Cold BM Pressure: _______

☐ Dry ☐ Humid ☐ Wet Allergen Levels: _______

☐ Sunny ☐ Cloudy

STRESS LEVELS

None	Low	Medium	High	Max	@$#%!

FOOD / DRINKS + NON-RELIEF MEDICATION / SUPPLEMENTS

item / meal	*time*	*meds / supplements*	*dose*	*time*

How many drinks?

water	① ② ③ ④ ⑤ ⑥ ⑦ ⑧ ⑨ ⑩
caffeine	① ② ③ ④ ⑤ ⑥ ⑦ ⑧ ⑨ ⑩
alcohol	① ② ③ ④ ⑤ ⑥ ⑦ ⑧ ⑨ ⑩

HORMONES

☐ Menstruating ☐ Menopause ☐ PMS ☐ N/A | other

COMPUTER USE / READING

☐ None ☐ Some ☐ A lot Total time:

☐ Sitting ☐ Standing ☐ Mixture Breaks every:

PHYSICAL ACTIVITY

☐ None ☐ Minimal ☐ Some ☐ Sweatin' ☐ I'm beat

DETAILS: ____________________

RELIEF MEASURES

☐ Medication ☐ Massage ☐ Sleep ☐ Exercise

☐ Water ☐ Cold/Ice ☐ Heat/Bath ☐ Other

DETAILS: ____________________

DID IT WORK? ☐ Nope ☐ A bit ☐ Mostly ☐ 100%

Notes

Entry #31

Date:________ **M T W T F S S**

START:		END:		DURATION:	

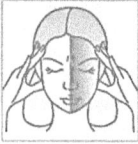

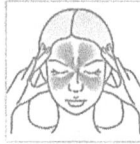

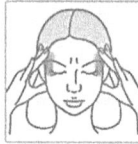

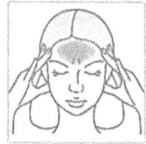

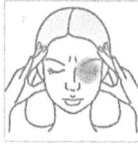

MIGRAINE CLUSTER SINUS TMJ TENSION

PAIN LEVEL

1	2	3	4	5	6	7	8	9	10

Not too bad. *Well, I'm not enjoying this.* *Make it stop!*

DETAILED DESCRIPTION

☐ Constant ☐ Squeezing ☐ Throbbing ☐ Pounding
☐ Dull aching ☐ Burning ☐ Sharp ☐ Debilitating

Other:________________________________

ONSET

☐ Slow ☐ Average ☐ Rapid ☐ Sudden

WHERE DOES IT HURT, EXACTLY?

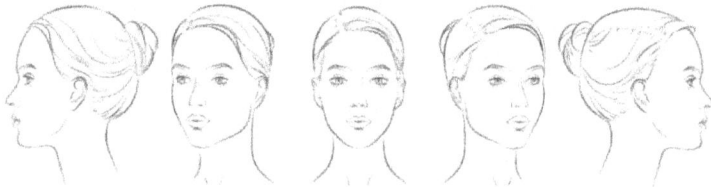

OTHER SYMPTOMS

☐ Lightheaded ☐ Dizziness ☐ Confusion
☐ Light sensitivity ☐ Sound sensitivity ☐ Auras
☐ Muscle stiffness ☐ Muscle burning ☐ Muscle aches

HOW ARE YOU FEELING OVERALL?

		Feeling sick?
Mood	① ② ③ ④ ⑤ ⑥ ⑦ ⑧ ⑨ ⑩	☐ Nope!
Energy levels	① ② ③ ④ ⑤ ⑥ ⑦ ⑧ ⑨ ⑩	☐ Yes...
Mental clarity	① ② ③ ④ ⑤ ⑥ ⑦ ⑧ ⑨ ⑩	

☐ Nausea ☐ Diarrhea ☐ Vomiting ☐ Sore throat
☐ Congestion ☐ Coughing ☐ Chills ☐ Fever

Other symptoms: ________________________

LAST NIGHT'S SLEEP

Hours of Sleep: ______________ Sleep Quality: ① ② ③ ④ ⑤

WEATHER

☐ Hot ☐ Mild ☐ Cold BM Pressure: _______

☐ Dry ☐ Humid ☐ Wet Allergen Levels: _______

☐ Sunny ☐ Cloudy

STRESS LEVELS

None	Low	Medium	High	Max	@$#%!

FOOD / DRINKS + NON-RELIEF MEDICATION / SUPPLEMENTS

item / meal	*time*	*meds / supplements*	*dose*	*time*

How many drinks?

water	→	① ② ③ ④ ⑤ ⑥ ⑦ ⑧ ⑨ ⑩
caffeine	→	① ② ③ ④ ⑤ ⑥ ⑦ ⑧ ⑨ ⑩
alcohol	→	① ② ③ ④ ⑤ ⑥ ⑦ ⑧ ⑨ ⑩

HORMONES

☐ Menstruating ☐ Menopause ☐ PMS ☐ N/A | other

COMPUTER USE / READING

☐ None ☐ Some ☐ A lot Total time: ☐

☐ Sitting ☐ Standing ☐ Mixture Breaks every: ☐

PHYSICAL ACTIVITY

☐ None ☐ Minimal ☐ Some ☐ Sweatin' ☐ I'm beat

DETAILS: ____

RELIEF MEASURES

☐ Medication ☐ Massage ☐ Sleep ☐ Exercise

☐ Water ☐ Cold/Ice ☐ Heat/Bath ☐ Other

DETAILS: ____

DID IT WORK? ☐ Nope ☐ A bit ☐ Mostly ☐ 100%

Notes

Entry #32

Date:________ M T W T F S S

START: END: DURATION:

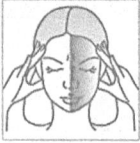

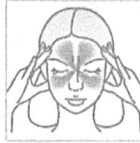

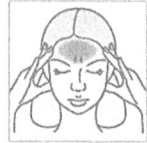

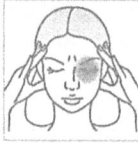

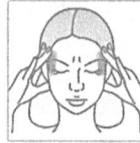

MIGRAINE CLUSTER SINUS TMJ TENSION

PAIN LEVEL

1	2	3	4	5	6	7	8	9	10

Not too bad. *Well, I'm not enjoying this.* *Make it stop!*

DETAILED DESCRIPTION

☐ Constant ☐ Squeezing ☐ Throbbing ☐ Pounding
☐ Dull aching ☐ Burning ☐ Sharp ☐ Debilitating

Other:

ONSET

☐ Slow ☐ Average ☐ Rapid ☐ Sudden

WHERE DOES IT HURT, EXACTLY?

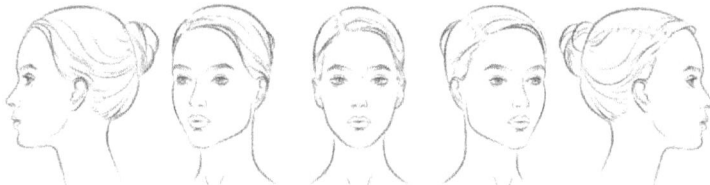

OTHER SYMPTOMS

☐ Lightheaded ☐ Dizziness ☐ Confusion
☐ Light sensitivity ☐ Sound sensitivity ☐ Auras
☐ Muscle stiffness ☐ Muscle burning ☐ Muscle aches

HOW ARE YOU FEELING OVERALL?

Mood	1	2	3	4	5	6	7	8	9	10
Energy levels	1	2	3	4	5	6	7	8	9	10
Mental clarity	1	2	3	4	5	6	7	8	9	10

Feeling sick?

☐ Nope!
☐ Yes...

☐ Nausea ☐ Diarrhea ☐ Vomiting ☐ Sore throat
☐ Congestion ☐ Coughing ☐ Chills ☐ Fever

Other symptoms:

LAST NIGHT'S SLEEP

Hours of Sleep: ____________ Sleep Quality: ① ② ③ ④ ⑤

WEATHER

☐ Hot ☐ Mild ☐ Cold BM Pressure: ______

☐ Dry ☐ Humid ☐ Wet Allergen Levels: ______

☐ Sunny ☐ Cloudy

STRESS LEVELS

None	Low	Medium	High	Max	@$#%!

FOOD / DRINKS + NON-RELIEF MEDICATION / SUPPLEMENTS

item / meal	*time*	*meds / supplements*	*dose*	*time*

How many drinks?

water	① ② ③ ④ ⑤ ⑥ ⑦ ⑧ ⑨ ⑩
caffeine	① ② ③ ④ ⑤ ⑥ ⑦ ⑧ ⑨ ⑩
alcohol	① ② ③ ④ ⑤ ⑥ ⑦ ⑧ ⑨ ⑩

HORMONES

☐ Menstruating ☐ Menopause ☐ PMS ☐ N/A | other

COMPUTER USE / READING

☐ None ☐ Some ☐ A lot Total time:

☐ Sitting ☐ Standing ☐ Mixture Breaks every:

PHYSICAL ACTIVITY

☐ None ☐ Minimal ☐ Some ☐ Sweatin' ☐ I'm beat

DETAILS: ______________________________

RELIEF MEASURES

☐ Medication ☐ Massage ☐ Sleep ☐ Exercise

☐ Water ☐ Cold/Ice ☐ Heat/Bath ☐ Other

DETAILS: ______________________________

DID IT WORK? ☐ Nope ☐ A bit ☐ Mostly ☐ 100%

Notes

Entry #33

Date:________ M T W T F S S

START:		END:		DURATION:	

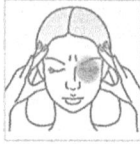

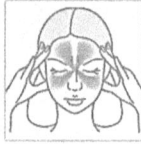

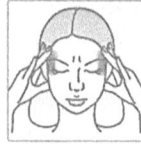

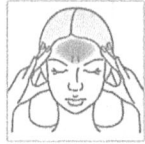

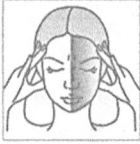

MIGRAINE CLUSTER SINUS TMJ TENSION

PAIN LEVEL

1	2	3	4	5	6	7	8	9	10

Not too bad. *Well, I'm not enjoying this.* *Make it stop!*

DETAILED DESCRIPTION

☐ Constant ☐ Squeezing ☐ Throbbing ☐ Pounding
☐ Dull aching ☐ Burning ☐ Sharp ☐ Debilitating

Other:______________________________

ONSET

☐ Slow ☐ Average ☐ Rapid ☐ Sudden

WHERE DOES IT HURT, EXACTLY?

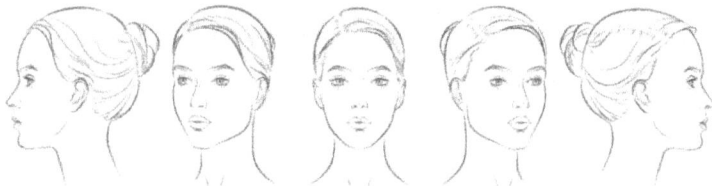

OTHER SYMPTOMS

☐ Lightheaded ☐ Dizziness ☐ Confusion
☐ Light sensitivity ☐ Sound sensitivity ☐ Auras
☐ Muscle stiffness ☐ Muscle burning ☐ Muscle aches

HOW ARE YOU FEELING OVERALL?

Mood	1	2	3	4	5	6	7	8	9	10
Energy levels	1	2	3	4	5	6	7	8	9	10
Mental clarity	1	2	3	4	5	6	7	8	9	10

Feeling sick?

☐ Nope!
☐ Yes…

☐ Nausea ☐ Diarrhea ☐ Vomiting ☐ Sore throat
☐ Congestion ☐ Coughing ☐ Chills ☐ Fever

Other symptoms: ______________________________

LAST NIGHT'S SLEEP

Hours of Sleep: ____________ Sleep Quality: ① ② ③ ④ ⑤

WEATHER

☐ Hot ☐ Mild ☐ Cold BM Pressure: ______

☐ Dry ☐ Humid ☐ Wet Allergen Levels: ______

☐ Sunny ☐ Cloudy

STRESS LEVELS

None	Low	Medium	High	Max	@$#%!

FOOD / DRINKS + NON-RELIEF MEDICATION / SUPPLEMENTS

item / meal	*time*	*meds / supplements*	*dose*	*time*

How many drinks?

water	① ② ③ ④ ⑤ ⑥ ⑦ ⑧ ⑨ ⑩
caffeine	① ② ③ ④ ⑤ ⑥ ⑦ ⑧ ⑨ ⑩
alcohol	① ② ③ ④ ⑤ ⑥ ⑦ ⑧ ⑨ ⑩

HORMONES

☐ Menstruating ☐ Menopause ☐ PMS ☐ N/A | other

COMPUTER USE / READING

☐ None ☐ Some ☐ A lot Total time:

☐ Sitting ☐ Standing ☐ Mixture Breaks every:

PHYSICAL ACTIVITY

☐ None ☐ Minimal ☐ Some ☐ Sweatin' ☐ I'm beat

DETAILS: ______________________________

RELIEF MEASURES

☐ Medication ☐ Massage ☐ Sleep ☐ Exercise

☐ Water ☐ Cold/Ice ☐ Heat/Bath ☐ Other

DETAILS: ______________________________

DID IT WORK? ☐ Nope ☐ A bit ☐ Mostly ☐ 100%

Notes

Entry #34

Date:________ M T W T F S S

START:		END:		DURATION:	

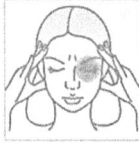

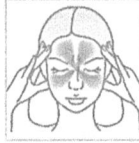

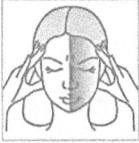

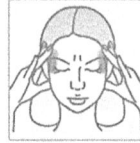

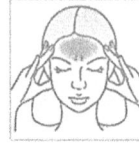

MIGRAINE CLUSTER SINUS TMJ TENSION

PAIN LEVEL

1	2	3	4	5	6	7	8	9	10

Not too bad. *Well, I'm not enjoying this.* *Make it stop!*

DETAILED DESCRIPTION

☐ Constant ☐ Squeezing ☐ Throbbing ☐ Pounding
☐ Dull aching ☐ Burning ☐ Sharp ☐ Debilitating

Other:________________________________

ONSET

☐ Slow ☐ Average ☐ Rapid ☐ Sudden

WHERE DOES IT HURT, EXACTLY?

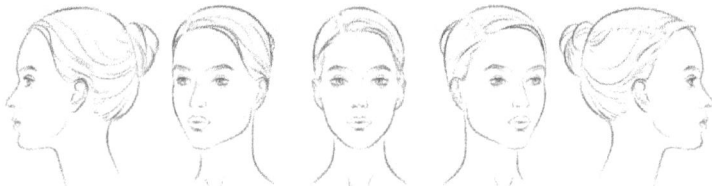

OTHER SYMPTOMS

☐ Lightheaded ☐ Dizziness ☐ Confusion
☐ Light sensitivity ☐ Sound sensitivity ☐ Auras
☐ Muscle stiffness ☐ Muscle burning ☐ Muscle aches

HOW ARE YOU FEELING OVERALL?

Mood	1	2	3	4	5	6	7	8	9	10
Energy levels	1	2	3	4	5	6	7	8	9	10
Mental clarity	1	2	3	4	5	6	7	8	9	10

Feeling sick?

☐ Nope!
☐ Yes...

☐ Nausea ☐ Diarrhea ☐ Vomiting ☐ Sore throat
☐ Congestion ☐ Coughing ☐ Chills ☐ Fever

Other symptoms:________________________________

LAST NIGHT'S SLEEP

Hours of Sleep: ____________ Sleep Quality: ① ② ③ ④ ⑤

WEATHER

☐ Hot ☐ Mild ☐ Cold BM Pressure: ______

☐ Dry ☐ Humid ☐ Wet Allergen Levels: ______

☐ Sunny ☐ Cloudy

STRESS LEVELS

None	Low	Medium	High	Max	@$#%!

FOOD / DRINKS + NON-RELIEF MEDICATION / SUPPLEMENTS

item / meal	*time*	*meds / supplements*	*dose*	*time*

How many drinks?

water	→	① ② ③ ④ ⑤ ⑥ ⑦ ⑧ ⑨ ⑩
caffeine	→	① ② ③ ④ ⑤ ⑥ ⑦ ⑧ ⑨ ⑩
alcohol	→	① ② ③ ④ ⑤ ⑥ ⑦ ⑧ ⑨ ⑩

HORMONES

☐ Menstruating ☐ Menopause ☐ PMS ☐ N/A | other

COMPUTER USE / READING

☐ None ☐ Some ☐ A lot Total time:

☐ Sitting ☐ Standing ☐ Mixture Breaks every:

PHYSICAL ACTIVITY

☐ None ☐ Minimal ☐ Some ☐ Sweatin' ☐ I'm beat

DETAILS: ______________________________

RELIEF MEASURES

☐ Medication ☐ Massage ☐ Sleep ☐ Exercise

☐ Water ☐ Cold/Ice ☐ Heat/Bath ☐ Other

DETAILS: ______________________________

DID IT WORK? ☐ Nope ☐ A bit ☐ Mostly ☐ 100%

Notes

Entry #35

Date:________ M T W T F S S

START:		END:		DURATION:	

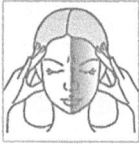

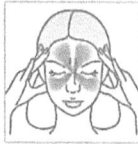

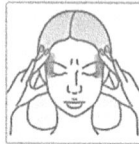

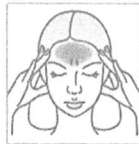

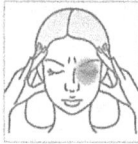

MIGRAINE CLUSTER SINUS TMJ TENSION

PAIN LEVEL

1	2	3	4	5	6	7	8	9	10

Not too bad. *Well, I'm not enjoying this.* *Make it stop!*

DETAILED DESCRIPTION

☐ Constant ☐ Squeezing ☐ Throbbing ☐ Pounding
☐ Dull aching ☐ Burning ☐ Sharp ☐ Debilitating

Other:______________________________

ONSET

☐ Slow ☐ Average ☐ Rapid ☐ Sudden

WHERE DOES IT HURT, EXACTLY?

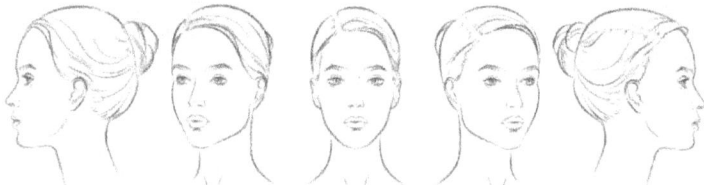

OTHER SYMPTOMS

☐ Lightheaded ☐ Dizziness ☐ Confusion
☐ Light sensitivity ☐ Sound sensitivity ☐ Auras
☐ Muscle stiffness ☐ Muscle burning ☐ Muscle aches

HOW ARE YOU FEELING OVERALL?

Mood	1	2	3	4	5	6	7	8	9	10
Energy levels	1	2	3	4	5	6	7	8	9	10
Mental clarity	1	2	3	4	5	6	7	8	9	10

Feeling sick?

☐ Nope!
☐ Yes...

☐ Nausea ☐ Diarrhea ☐ Vomiting ☐ Sore throat
☐ Congestion ☐ Coughing ☐ Chills ☐ Fever

Other symptoms: ______________________________

LAST NIGHT'S SLEEP

Hours of Sleep: ____________ Sleep Quality: ① ② ③ ④ ⑤

WEATHER

☐ Hot ☐ Mild ☐ Cold BM Pressure: ______

☐ Dry ☐ Humid ☐ Wet Allergen Levels: ______

☐ Sunny ☐ Cloudy

STRESS LEVELS

None	Low	Medium	High	Max	@$#%!

FOOD / DRINKS + NON-RELIEF MEDICATION / SUPPLEMENTS

item / meal	*time*	*meds / supplements*	*dose*	*time*

How many drinks?

water	① ② ③ ④ ⑤ ⑥ ⑦ ⑧ ⑨ ⑩
caffeine	① ② ③ ④ ⑤ ⑥ ⑦ ⑧ ⑨ ⑩
alcohol	① ② ③ ④ ⑤ ⑥ ⑦ ⑧ ⑨ ⑩

HORMONES

☐ Menstruating ☐ Menopause ☐ PMS ☐ N/A | other

COMPUTER USE / READING

☐ None ☐ Some ☐ A lot Total time:

☐ Sitting ☐ Standing ☐ Mixture Breaks every:

PHYSICAL ACTIVITY

☐ None ☐ Minimal ☐ Some ☐ Sweatin' ☐ I'm beat

DETAILS: ________________________________

RELIEF MEASURES

☐ Medication ☐ Massage ☐ Sleep ☐ Exercise

☐ Water ☐ Cold/Ice ☐ Heat/Bath ☐ Other

DETAILS: ________________________________

DID IT WORK? ☐ Nope ☐ A bit ☐ Mostly ☐ 100%

Notes

Entry #36

Date:________ M T W T F S S

START:		END:		DURATION:	

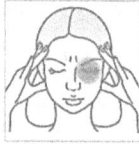

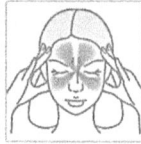

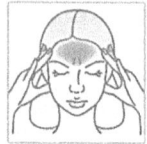

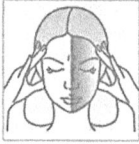

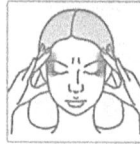

MIGRAINE CLUSTER SINUS TMJ TENSION

PAIN LEVEL

1	2	3	4	5	6	7	8	9	10

Not too bad. *Well, I'm not enjoying this.* *Make it stop!*

DETAILED DESCRIPTION

☐ Constant ☐ Squeezing ☐ Throbbing ☐ Pounding
☐ Dull aching ☐ Burning ☐ Sharp ☐ Debilitating

Other:____________________

ONSET

☐ Slow ☐ Average ☐ Rapid ☐ Sudden

WHERE DOES IT HURT, EXACTLY?

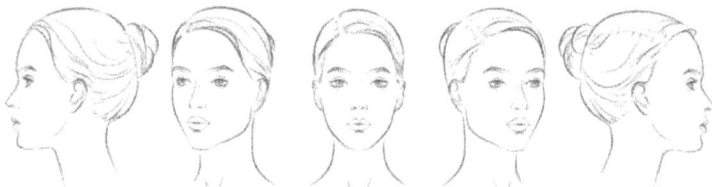

OTHER SYMPTOMS

☐ Lightheaded ☐ Dizziness ☐ Confusion
☐ Light sensitivity ☐ Sound sensitivity ☐ Auras
☐ Muscle stiffness ☐ Muscle burning ☐ Muscle aches

HOW ARE YOU FEELING OVERALL?

Mood	1	2	3	4	5	6	7	8	9	10
Energy levels	1	2	3	4	5	6	7	8	9	10
Mental clarity	1	2	3	4	5	6	7	8	9	10

Feeling sick?

☐ Nope!
☐ Yes...

☐ Nausea ☐ Diarrhea ☐ Vomiting ☐ Sore throat
☐ Congestion ☐ Coughing ☐ Chills ☐ Fever

Other symptoms: ____________________

LAST NIGHT'S SLEEP

Hours of Sleep: ____________ Sleep Quality: ① ② ③ ④ ⑤

WEATHER

☐ Hot ☐ Mild ☐ Cold BM Pressure: ______

☐ Dry ☐ Humid ☐ Wet Allergen Levels: ______

☐ Sunny ☐ Cloudy

STRESS LEVELS

None	Low	Medium	High	Max	@$#%!

FOOD / DRINKS + NON-RELIEF MEDICATION / SUPPLEMENTS

item / meal	*time*	*meds / supplements*	*dose*	*time*
		How many drinks?		

water	→	① ② ③ ④ ⑤ ⑥ ⑦ ⑧ ⑨ ⑩
caffeine	→	① ② ③ ④ ⑤ ⑥ ⑦ ⑧ ⑨ ⑩
alcohol	→	① ② ③ ④ ⑤ ⑥ ⑦ ⑧ ⑨ ⑩

HORMONES

☐ Menstruating ☐ Menopause ☐ PMS ☐ N/A | other

COMPUTER USE / READING

☐ None ☐ Some ☐ A lot Total time: ______

☐ Sitting ☐ Standing ☐ Mixture Breaks every: ______

PHYSICAL ACTIVITY

☐ None ☐ Minimal ☐ Some ☐ Sweatin' ☐ I'm beat

DETAILS: ____

RELIEF MEASURES

☐ Medication ☐ Massage ☐ Sleep ☐ Exercise

☐ Water ☐ Cold/Ice ☐ Heat/Bath ☐ Other

DETAILS: ____

DID IT WORK? ☐ Nope ☐ A bit ☐ Mostly ☐ 100%

Notes

Entry #37

Date:________ MTWTFSS

START:		END:		DURATION:	

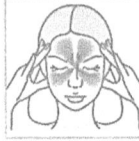

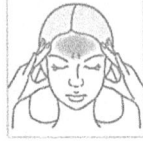

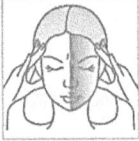

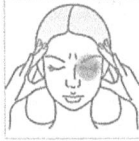

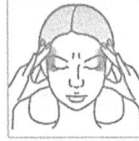

MIGRAINE CLUSTER SINUS TMJ TENSION

PAIN LEVEL

1	2	3	4	5	6	7	8	9	10

Not too bad. *Well, I'm not enjoying this.* *Make it stop!*

DETAILED DESCRIPTION

☐ Constant ☐ Squeezing ☐ Throbbing ☐ Pounding
☐ Dull aching ☐ Burning ☐ Sharp ☐ Debilitating

Other:______________________________

ONSET

☐ Slow ☐ Average ☐ Rapid ☐ Sudden

WHERE DOES IT HURT, EXACTLY?

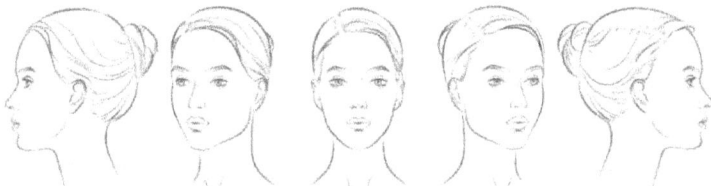

OTHER SYMPTOMS

☐ Lightheaded ☐ Dizziness ☐ Confusion
☐ Light sensitivity ☐ Sound sensitivity ☐ Auras
☐ Muscle stiffness ☐ Muscle burning ☐ Muscle aches

HOW ARE YOU FEELING OVERALL? Feeling sick?

Mood	① ② ③ ④ ⑤ ⑥ ⑦ ⑧ ⑨ ⑩	☐ Nope!
Energy levels	① ② ③ ④ ⑤ ⑥ ⑦ ⑧ ⑨ ⑩	☐ Yes...
Mental clarity	① ② ③ ④ ⑤ ⑥ ⑦ ⑧ ⑨ ⑩	

☐ Nausea ☐ Diarrhea ☐ Vomiting ☐ Sore throat
☐ Congestion ☐ Coughing ☐ Chills ☐ Fever

Other symptoms: ______________________________

LAST NIGHT'S SLEEP

Hours of Sleep: ____________ Sleep Quality: ① ② ③ ④ ⑤

WEATHER

☐ Hot ☐ Mild ☐ Cold BM Pressure: ______

☐ Dry ☐ Humid ☐ Wet Allergen Levels: ______

☐ Sunny ☐ Cloudy

STRESS LEVELS

None	Low	Medium	High	Max	@$#%!

FOOD / DRINKS + NON-RELIEF MEDICATION / SUPPLEMENTS

item / meal	*time*	*meds / supplements*	*dose*	*time*
		How many drinks?		

water	→	① ② ③ ④ ⑤ ⑥ ⑦ ⑧ ⑨ ⑩
caffeine	→	① ② ③ ④ ⑤ ⑥ ⑦ ⑧ ⑨ ⑩
alcohol	→	① ② ③ ④ ⑤ ⑥ ⑦ ⑧ ⑨ ⑩

HORMONES

☐ Menstruating ☐ Menopause ☐ PMS ☐ N/A | other

COMPUTER USE / READING

☐ None ☐ Some ☐ A lot Total time: ______

☐ Sitting ☐ Standing ☐ Mixture Breaks every: ______

PHYSICAL ACTIVITY

☐ None ☐ Minimal ☐ Some ☐ Sweatin' ☐ I'm beat

DETAILS: ____

RELIEF MEASURES

☐ Medication ☐ Massage ☐ Sleep ☐ Exercise

☐ Water ☐ Cold/Ice ☐ Heat/Bath ☐ Other

DETAILS: ____

DID IT WORK? ☐ Nope ☐ A bit ☐ Mostly ☐ 100%

Notes

Entry #38

Date:________ M T W T F S S

START:		END:		DURATION:	

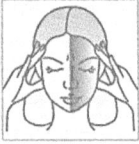

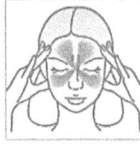

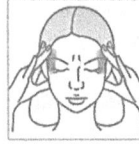

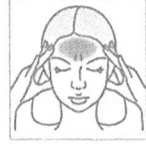

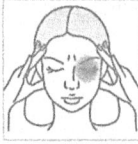

MIGRAINE CLUSTER SINUS TMJ TENSION

PAIN LEVEL

1	2	3	4	5	6	7	8	9	10

Not too bad. *Well, I'm not enjoying this.* *Make it stop!*

DETAILED DESCRIPTION

☐ Constant ☐ Squeezing ☐ Throbbing ☐ Pounding
☐ Dull aching ☐ Burning ☐ Sharp ☐ Debilitating

Other:______________________________

ONSET

☐ Slow ☐ Average ☐ Rapid ☐ Sudden

WHERE DOES IT HURT, EXACTLY?

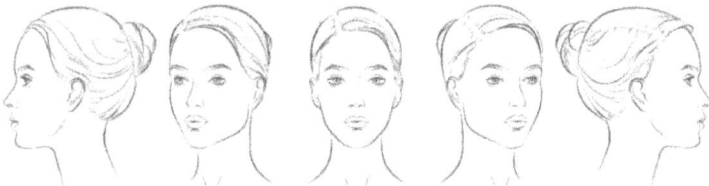

OTHER SYMPTOMS

☐ Lightheaded ☐ Dizziness ☐ Confusion
☐ Light sensitivity ☐ Sound sensitivity ☐ Auras
☐ Muscle stiffness ☐ Muscle burning ☐ Muscle aches

HOW ARE YOU FEELING OVERALL?

		Feeling sick?
Mood	① ② ③ ④ ⑤ ⑥ ⑦ ⑧ ⑨ ⑩	☐ Nope!
Energy levels	① ② ③ ④ ⑤ ⑥ ⑦ ⑧ ⑨ ⑩	☐ Yes...
Mental clarity	① ② ③ ④ ⑤ ⑥ ⑦ ⑧ ⑨ ⑩	

☐ Nausea ☐ Diarrhea ☐ Vomiting ☐ Sore throat
☐ Congestion ☐ Coughing ☐ Chills ☐ Fever

Other symptoms: ______________________________

LAST NIGHT'S SLEEP

Hours of Sleep: ____________ Sleep Quality: ① ② ③ ④ ⑤

WEATHER

☐ Hot ☐ Mild ☐ Cold BM Pressure: ______

☐ Dry ☐ Humid ☐ Wet Allergen Levels: ______

☐ Sunny ☐ Cloudy

STRESS LEVELS

None	Low	Medium	High	Max	@$#%!

FOOD / DRINKS + NON-RELIEF MEDICATION / SUPPLEMENTS

item / meal	*time*	*meds / supplements*	*dose*	*time*
		How many drinks?		

water	→	① ② ③ ④ ⑤ ⑥ ⑦ ⑧ ⑨ ⑩
caffeine	→	① ② ③ ④ ⑤ ⑥ ⑦ ⑧ ⑨ ⑩
alcohol	→	① ② ③ ④ ⑤ ⑥ ⑦ ⑧ ⑨ ⑩

HORMONES

☐ Menstruating ☐ Menopause ☐ PMS ☐ N/A | other

COMPUTER USE / READING

☐ None ☐ Some ☐ A lot Total time: ☐

☐ Sitting ☐ Standing ☐ Mixture Breaks every: ☐

PHYSICAL ACTIVITY

☐ None ☐ Minimal ☐ Some ☐ Sweatin' ☐ I'm beat

DETAILS: ______________________________

RELIEF MEASURES

☐ Medication ☐ Massage ☐ Sleep ☐ Exercise

☐ Water ☐ Cold/Ice ☐ Heat/Bath ☐ Other

DETAILS: ______________________________

DID IT WORK? ☐ Nope ☐ A bit ☐ Mostly ☐ 100%

Notes

Entry #39

Date:_______ M T W T F S S

START:		END:		DURATION:	

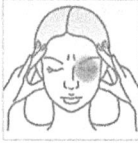

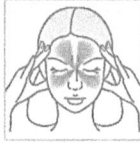

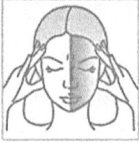

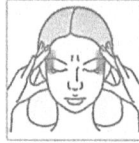

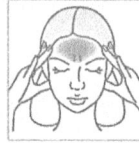

MIGRAINE CLUSTER SINUS TMJ TENSION

PAIN LEVEL

1	2	3	4	5	6	7	8	9	10

Not too bad. *Well, I'm not enjoying this.* *Make it stop!*

DETAILED DESCRIPTION

☐ Constant ☐ Squeezing ☐ Throbbing ☐ Pounding
☐ Dull aching ☐ Burning ☐ Sharp ☐ Debilitating

Other:____

ONSET

☐ Slow ☐ Average ☐ Rapid ☐ Sudden

WHERE DOES IT HURT, EXACTLY?

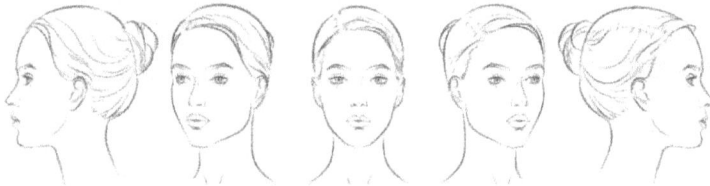

OTHER SYMPTOMS

☐ Lightheaded ☐ Dizziness ☐ Confusion
☐ Light sensitivity ☐ Sound sensitivity ☐ Auras
☐ Muscle stiffness ☐ Muscle burning ☐ Muscle aches

HOW ARE YOU FEELING OVERALL?

		Feeling sick?
Mood	① ② ③ ④ ⑤ ⑥ ⑦ ⑧ ⑨ ⑩	☐ Nope!
Energy levels	① ② ③ ④ ⑤ ⑥ ⑦ ⑧ ⑨ ⑩	☐ Yes...
Mental clarity	① ② ③ ④ ⑤ ⑥ ⑦ ⑧ ⑨ ⑩	

☐ Nausea ☐ Diarrhea ☐ Vomiting ☐ Sore throat
☐ Congestion ☐ Coughing ☐ Chills ☐ Fever

Other symptoms: ______________________________________

LAST NIGHT'S SLEEP

Hours of Sleep: ______________ Sleep Quality: ① ② ③ ④ ⑤

WEATHER

☐ Hot ☐ Mild ☐ Cold BM Pressure: _______

☐ Dry ☐ Humid ☐ Wet Allergen Levels: _______

☐ Sunny ☐ Cloudy

STRESS LEVELS

None	Low	Medium	High	Max	@$#%!

FOOD / DRINKS + NON-RELIEF MEDICATION / SUPPLEMENTS

item / meal	*time*	*meds / supplements*	*dose*	*time*

How many drinks?

water	① ② ③ ④ ⑤ ⑥ ⑦ ⑧ ⑨ ⑩
caffeine	① ② ③ ④ ⑤ ⑥ ⑦ ⑧ ⑨ ⑩
alcohol	① ② ③ ④ ⑤ ⑥ ⑦ ⑧ ⑨ ⑩

HORMONES

☐ Menstruating ☐ Menopause ☐ PMS ☐ N/A | other

COMPUTER USE / READING

☐ None ☐ Some ☐ A lot Total time:

☐ Sitting ☐ Standing ☐ Mixture Breaks every:

PHYSICAL ACTIVITY

☐ None ☐ Minimal ☐ Some ☐ Sweatin' ☐ I'm beat

DETAILS: ____

RELIEF MEASURES

☐ Medication ☐ Massage ☐ Sleep ☐ Exercise

☐ Water ☐ Cold/Ice ☐ Heat/Bath ☐ Other

DETAILS: ____

DID IT WORK? ☐ Nope ☐ A bit ☐ Mostly ☐ 100%

Notes

Entry #40

Date:________ M T W T F S S

START:		END:		DURATION:	

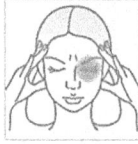

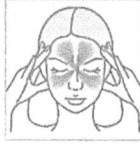

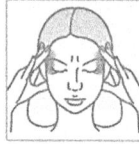

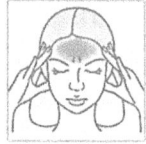

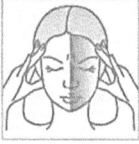

MIGRAINE CLUSTER SINUS TMJ TENSION

PAIN LEVEL

1	2	3	4	5	6	7	8	9	10

Not too bad. *Well, I'm not enjoying this.* *Make it stop!*

DETAILED DESCRIPTION

☐ Constant ☐ Squeezing ☐ Throbbing ☐ Pounding
☐ Dull aching ☐ Burning ☐ Sharp ☐ Debilitating

Other:______________________________

ONSET

☐ Slow ☐ Average ☐ Rapid ☐ Sudden

WHERE DOES IT HURT, EXACTLY?

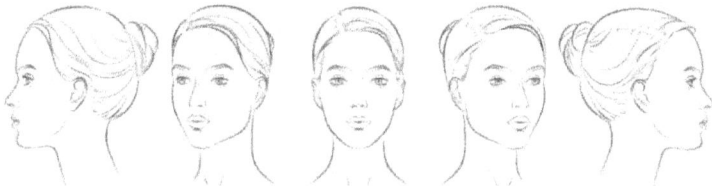

OTHER SYMPTOMS

☐ Lightheaded ☐ Dizziness ☐ Confusion
☐ Light sensitivity ☐ Sound sensitivity ☐ Auras
☐ Muscle stiffness ☐ Muscle burning ☐ Muscle aches

HOW ARE YOU FEELING OVERALL?

Mood	1	2	3	4	5	6	7	8	9	10
Energy levels	1	2	3	4	5	6	7	8	9	10
Mental clarity	1	2	3	4	5	6	7	8	9	10

Feeling sick?

☐ Nope!
☐ Yes...

☐ Nausea ☐ Diarrhea ☐ Vomiting ☐ Sore throat
☐ Congestion ☐ Coughing ☐ Chills ☐ Fever

Other symptoms: ______________________________

LAST NIGHT'S SLEEP

Hours of Sleep: ______________ Sleep Quality: ① ② ③ ④ ⑤

WEATHER

☐ Hot ☐ Mild ☐ Cold BM Pressure: _______

☐ Dry ☐ Humid ☐ Wet Allergen Levels: _______

☐ Sunny ☐ Cloudy

STRESS LEVELS

None	Low	Medium	High	Max	@$#%!

FOOD / DRINKS + NON-RELIEF MEDICATION / SUPPLEMENTS

item / meal	time	meds / supplements	dose	time

How many drinks?

water	① ② ③ ④ ⑤ ⑥ ⑦ ⑧ ⑨ ⑩
caffeine	① ② ③ ④ ⑤ ⑥ ⑦ ⑧ ⑨ ⑩
alcohol	① ② ③ ④ ⑤ ⑥ ⑦ ⑧ ⑨ ⑩

HORMONES

☐ Menstruating ☐ Menopause ☐ PMS ☐ N/A | other

COMPUTER USE / READING

☐ None ☐ Some ☐ A lot Total time:

☐ Sitting ☐ Standing ☐ Mixture Breaks every:

PHYSICAL ACTIVITY

☐ None ☐ Minimal ☐ Some ☐ Sweatin' ☐ I'm beat

DETAILS: ______________________________

RELIEF MEASURES

☐ Medication ☐ Massage ☐ Sleep ☐ Exercise

☐ Water ☐ Cold/Ice ☐ Heat/Bath ☐ Other

DETAILS: ______________________________

DID IT WORK? ☐ Nope ☐ A bit ☐ Mostly ☐ 100%

Notes

Entry #41

Date:________ M T W T F S S

START:		END:		DURATION:	

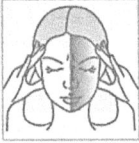

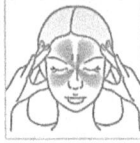

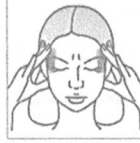

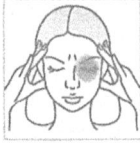

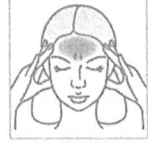

MIGRAINE CLUSTER SINUS TMJ TENSION

PAIN LEVEL

1	2	3	4	5	6	7	8	9	10

Not too bad. *Well, I'm not enjoying this.* *Make it stop!*

DETAILED DESCRIPTION

☐ Constant ☐ Squeezing ☐ Throbbing ☐ Pounding
☐ Dull aching ☐ Burning ☐ Sharp ☐ Debilitating

Other:______________________________

ONSET

☐ Slow ☐ Average ☐ Rapid ☐ Sudden

WHERE DOES IT HURT, EXACTLY?

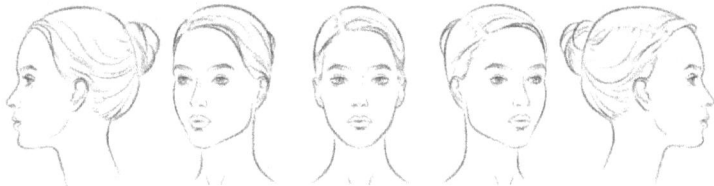

OTHER SYMPTOMS

☐ Lightheaded ☐ Dizziness ☐ Confusion
☐ Light sensitivity ☐ Sound sensitivity ☐ Auras
☐ Muscle stiffness ☐ Muscle burning ☐ Muscle aches

HOW ARE YOU FEELING OVERALL?

Mood	1	2	3	4	5	6	7	8	9	10
Energy levels	1	2	3	4	5	6	7	8	9	10
Mental clarity	1	2	3	4	5	6	7	8	9	10

Feeling sick?

☐ Nope!
☐ Yes...

☐ Nausea ☐ Diarrhea ☐ Vomiting ☐ Sore throat
☐ Congestion ☐ Coughing ☐ Chills ☐ Fever

Other symptoms: ______________________________

LAST NIGHT'S SLEEP

Hours of Sleep: ____________ Sleep Quality: ① ② ③ ④ ⑤

WEATHER

☐ Hot ☐ Mild ☐ Cold BM Pressure: ______

☐ Dry ☐ Humid ☐ Wet Allergen Levels: ______

☐ Sunny ☐ Cloudy

STRESS LEVELS

None	Low	Medium	High	Max	@$#%!

FOOD / DRINKS + NON-RELIEF MEDICATION / SUPPLEMENTS

item / meal	*time*	*meds / supplements*	*dose*	*time*

How many drinks?

water →	1	2	3	4	5	6	7	8	9	10
caffeine →	1	2	3	4	5	6	7	8	9	10
alcohol →	1	2	3	4	5	6	7	8	9	10

HORMONES

☐ Menstruating ☐ Menopause ☐ PMS ☐ N/A | other

COMPUTER USE / READING

☐ None ☐ Some ☐ A lot Total time: ______

☐ Sitting ☐ Standing ☐ Mixture Breaks every: ______

PHYSICAL ACTIVITY

☐ None ☐ Minimal ☐ Some ☐ Sweatin' ☐ I'm beat

DETAILS: ____

RELIEF MEASURES

☐ Medication ☐ Massage ☐ Sleep ☐ Exercise

☐ Water ☐ Cold/Ice ☐ Heat/Bath ☐ Other

DETAILS: ____

DID IT WORK? ☐ Nope ☐ A bit ☐ Mostly ☐ 100%

Notes

Entry #42

Date:________ M T W T F S S

START:		END:		DURATION:	

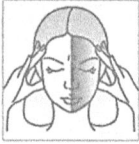

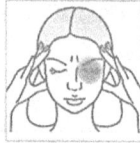

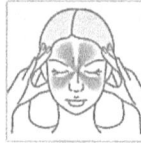

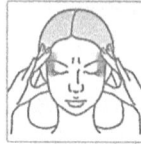

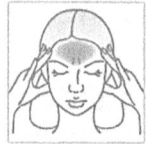

MIGRAINE CLUSTER SINUS TMJ TENSION

PAIN LEVEL

1	2	3	4	5	6	7	8	9	10

Not too bad. *Well, I'm not enjoying this.* *Make it stop!*

DETAILED DESCRIPTION

☐ Constant ☐ Squeezing ☐ Throbbing ☐ Pounding
☐ Dull aching ☐ Burning ☐ Sharp ☐ Debilitating

Other:______________________________

ONSET

☐ Slow ☐ Average ☐ Rapid ☐ Sudden

WHERE DOES IT HURT, EXACTLY?

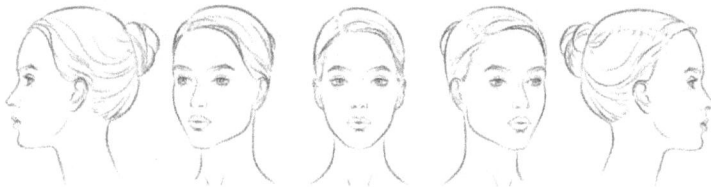

OTHER SYMPTOMS

☐ Lightheaded ☐ Dizziness ☐ Confusion
☐ Light sensitivity ☐ Sound sensitivity ☐ Auras
☐ Muscle stiffness ☐ Muscle burning ☐ Muscle aches

HOW ARE YOU FEELING OVERALL?

Mood	1	2	3	4	5	6	7	8	9	10
Energy levels	1	2	3	4	5	6	7	8	9	10
Mental clarity	1	2	3	4	5	6	7	8	9	10

Feeling sick?

☐ Nope!
☐ Yes...

☐ Nausea ☐ Diarrhea ☐ Vomiting ☐ Sore throat
☐ Congestion ☐ Coughing ☐ Chills ☐ Fever

Other symptoms: ______________________________

LAST NIGHT'S SLEEP

Hours of Sleep: ____________ Sleep Quality: ① ② ③ ④ ⑤

WEATHER

☐ Hot ☐ Mild ☐ Cold BM Pressure: ______
☐ Dry ☐ Humid ☐ Wet Allergen Levels: ______
☐ Sunny ☐ Cloudy

STRESS LEVELS

None	Low	Medium	High	Max	@$#%!

FOOD / DRINKS + NON-RELIEF MEDICATION / SUPPLEMENTS

item / meal	*time*	*meds / supplements*	*dose*	*time*

How many drinks?

water	① ② ③ ④ ⑤ ⑥ ⑦ ⑧ ⑨ ⑩
caffeine	① ② ③ ④ ⑤ ⑥ ⑦ ⑧ ⑨ ⑩
alcohol	① ② ③ ④ ⑤ ⑥ ⑦ ⑧ ⑨ ⑩

HORMONES

☐ Menstruating ☐ Menopause ☐ PMS ☐ N/A | other

COMPUTER USE / READING

☐ None ☐ Some ☐ A lot Total time: ______
☐ Sitting ☐ Standing ☐ Mixture Breaks every: ______

PHYSICAL ACTIVITY

☐ None ☐ Minimal ☐ Some ☐ Sweatin' ☐ I'm beat

DETAILS: ____________________

RELIEF MEASURES

☐ Medication ☐ Massage ☐ Sleep ☐ Exercise
☐ Water ☐ Cold/Ice ☐ Heat/Bath ☐ Other

DETAILS: ____________________

DID IT WORK? ☐ Nope ☐ A bit ☐ Mostly ☐ 100%

Notes

Entry #43

Date:________ M T W T F S S

START: END: DURATION:

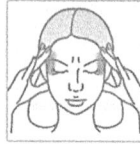

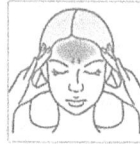

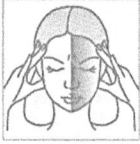

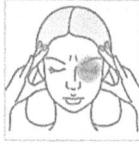

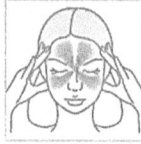

MIGRAINE CLUSTER SINUS TMJ TENSION

PAIN LEVEL

1	2	3	4	5	6	7	8	9	10

Not too bad. *Well, I'm not enjoying this.* *Make it stop!*

DETAILED DESCRIPTION

☐ Constant ☐ Squeezing ☐ Throbbing ☐ Pounding
☐ Dull aching ☐ Burning ☐ Sharp ☐ Debilitating

Other:____________________

ONSET

☐ Slow ☐ Average ☐ Rapid ☐ Sudden

WHERE DOES IT HURT, EXACTLY?

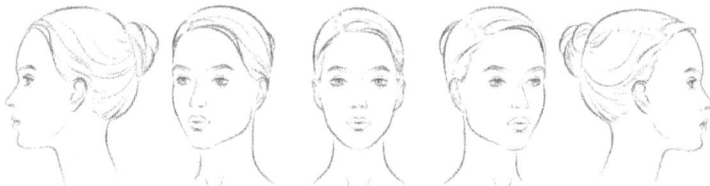

OTHER SYMPTOMS

☐ Lightheaded ☐ Dizziness ☐ Confusion
☐ Light sensitivity ☐ Sound sensitivity ☐ Auras
☐ Muscle stiffness ☐ Muscle burning ☐ Muscle aches

HOW ARE YOU FEELING OVERALL?

		Feeling sick?
Mood	① ② ③ ④ ⑤ ⑥ ⑦ ⑧ ⑨ ⑩	☐ Nope!
Energy levels	① ② ③ ④ ⑤ ⑥ ⑦ ⑧ ⑨ ⑩	☐ Yes…
Mental clarity	① ② ③ ④ ⑤ ⑥ ⑦ ⑧ ⑨ ⑩	

☐ Nausea ☐ Diarrhea ☐ Vomiting ☐ Sore throat
☐ Congestion ☐ Coughing ☐ Chills ☐ Fever

Other symptoms: ____________________

LAST NIGHT'S SLEEP

Hours of Sleep: ____________ Sleep Quality: ① ② ③ ④ ⑤

WEATHER

☐ Hot ☐ Mild ☐ Cold BM Pressure: ______

☐ Dry ☐ Humid ☐ Wet Allergen Levels: ______

☐ Sunny ☐ Cloudy

STRESS LEVELS

None	Low	Medium	High	Max	@$#%!

FOOD / DRINKS + NON-RELIEF MEDICATION / SUPPLEMENTS

item / meal	*time*	*meds / supplements*	*dose*	*time*

How many drinks?

water	① ② ③ ④ ⑤ ⑥ ⑦ ⑧ ⑨ ⑩
caffeine	① ② ③ ④ ⑤ ⑥ ⑦ ⑧ ⑨ ⑩
alcohol	① ② ③ ④ ⑤ ⑥ ⑦ ⑧ ⑨ ⑩

HORMONES

☐ Menstruating ☐ Menopause ☐ PMS ☐ N/A | other

COMPUTER USE / READING

☐ None ☐ Some ☐ A lot Total time: ______

☐ Sitting ☐ Standing ☐ Mixture Breaks every: ______

PHYSICAL ACTIVITY

☐ None ☐ Minimal ☐ Some ☐ Sweatin' ☐ I'm beat

DETAILS: ________________________________

RELIEF MEASURES

☐ Medication ☐ Massage ☐ Sleep ☐ Exercise

☐ Water ☐ Cold/Ice ☐ Heat/Bath ☐ Other

DETAILS: ________________________________

DID IT WORK? ☐ Nope ☐ A bit ☐ Mostly ☐ 100%

Notes

Entry #44

Date:________ **M T W T F S S**

START:		END:		DURATION:	

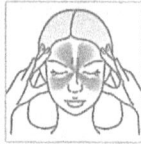

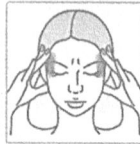

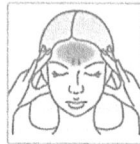

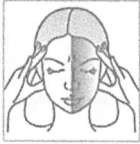

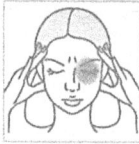

MIGRAINE CLUSTER SINUS TMJ TENSION

PAIN LEVEL

1	2	3	4	5	6	7	8	9	10

Not too bad. *Well, I'm not enjoying this.* *Make it stop!*

DETAILED DESCRIPTION

☐ Constant ☐ Squeezing ☐ Throbbing ☐ Pounding
☐ Dull aching ☐ Burning ☐ Sharp ☐ Debilitating

Other:____________________

ONSET

☐ Slow ☐ Average ☐ Rapid ☐ Sudden

WHERE DOES IT HURT, EXACTLY?

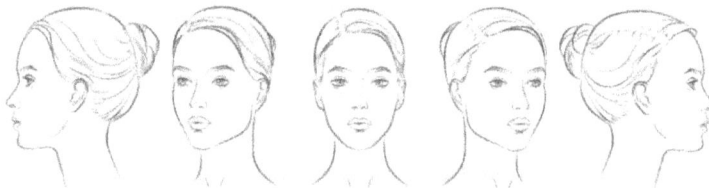

OTHER SYMPTOMS

☐ Lightheaded ☐ Dizziness ☐ Confusion
☐ Light sensitivity ☐ Sound sensitivity ☐ Auras
☐ Muscle stiffness ☐ Muscle burning ☐ Muscle aches

HOW ARE YOU FEELING OVERALL?

Mood	1	2	3	4	5	6	7	8	9	10
Energy levels	1	2	3	4	5	6	7	8	9	10
Mental clarity	1	2	3	4	5	6	7	8	9	10

Feeling sick?

☐ Nope!
☐ Yes...

☐ Nausea ☐ Diarrhea ☐ Vomiting ☐ Sore throat
☐ Congestion ☐ Coughing ☐ Chills ☐ Fever

Other symptoms: ____________________

LAST NIGHT'S SLEEP

Hours of Sleep: ____________ Sleep Quality: ① ② ③ ④ ⑤

WEATHER

☐ Hot ☐ Mild ☐ Cold BM Pressure: ______

☐ Dry ☐ Humid ☐ Wet Allergen Levels: ______

☐ Sunny ☐ Cloudy

STRESS LEVELS

None	Low	Medium	High	Max	@$#%!

FOOD / DRINKS + NON-RELIEF MEDICATION / SUPPLEMENTS

item / meal	*time*	*meds / supplements*	*dose*	*time*

How many drinks?

water	① ② ③ ④ ⑤ ⑥ ⑦ ⑧ ⑨ ⑩
caffeine	① ② ③ ④ ⑤ ⑥ ⑦ ⑧ ⑨ ⑩
alcohol	① ② ③ ④ ⑤ ⑥ ⑦ ⑧ ⑨ ⑩

HORMONES

☐ Menstruating ☐ Menopause ☐ PMS ☐ N/A | other

COMPUTER USE / READING

☐ None ☐ Some ☐ A lot Total time: ______

☐ Sitting ☐ Standing ☐ Mixture Breaks every: ______

PHYSICAL ACTIVITY

☐ None ☐ Minimal ☐ Some ☐ Sweatin' ☐ I'm beat

DETAILS: ____________________

RELIEF MEASURES

☐ Medication ☐ Massage ☐ Sleep ☐ Exercise

☐ Water ☐ Cold/Ice ☐ Heat/Bath ☐ Other

DETAILS: ____________________

DID IT WORK? ☐ Nope ☐ A bit ☐ Mostly ☐ 100%

Notes

Entry #45

Date:________

M T W T F S S

START:		END:		DURATION:	

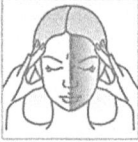

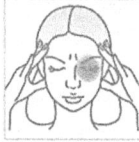

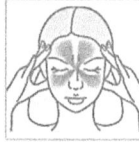

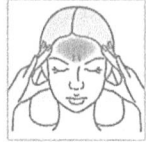

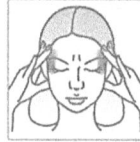

MIGRAINE CLUSTER SINUS TMJ TENSION

PAIN LEVEL

1	2	3	4	5	6	7	8	9	10

Not too bad. *Well, I'm not enjoying this.* *Make it stop!*

DETAILED DESCRIPTION

☐ Constant ☐ Squeezing ☐ Throbbing ☐ Pounding
☐ Dull aching ☐ Burning ☐ Sharp ☐ Debilitating

Other:________________________________

ONSET

☐ Slow ☐ Average ☐ Rapid ☐ Sudden

WHERE DOES IT HURT, EXACTLY?

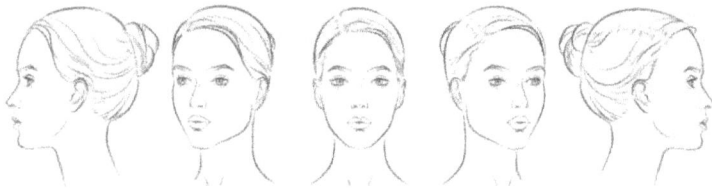

OTHER SYMPTOMS

☐ Lightheaded ☐ Dizziness ☐ Confusion
☐ Light sensitivity ☐ Sound sensitivity ☐ Auras
☐ Muscle stiffness ☐ Muscle burning ☐ Muscle aches

HOW ARE YOU FEELING OVERALL?

Mood	1	2	3	4	5	6	7	8	9	10
Energy levels	1	2	3	4	5	6	7	8	9	10
Mental clarity	1	2	3	4	5	6	7	8	9	10

Feeling sick?

☐ Nope!
☐ Yes...

☐ Nausea ☐ Diarrhea ☐ Vomiting ☐ Sore throat
☐ Congestion ☐ Coughing ☐ Chills ☐ Fever

Other symptoms:________________________________

LAST NIGHT'S SLEEP

Hours of Sleep: ____________ Sleep Quality: (1) (2) (3) (4) (5)

WEATHER

☐ Hot ☐ Mild ☐ Cold BM Pressure: ______

☐ Dry ☐ Humid ☐ Wet Allergen Levels: ______

☐ Sunny ☐ Cloudy

STRESS LEVELS

None	Low	Medium	High	Max	@$#%!

FOOD / DRINKS + NON-RELIEF MEDICATION / SUPPLEMENTS

item / meal	*time*	*meds / supplements*	*dose*	*time*

How many drinks?

water	(1) (2) (3) (4) (5) (6) (7) (8) (9) (10)
caffeine	(1) (2) (3) (4) (5) (6) (7) (8) (9) (10)
alcohol	(1) (2) (3) (4) (5) (6) (7) (8) (9) (10)

HORMONES

☐ Menstruating ☐ Menopause ☐ PMS ☐ N/A | other

COMPUTER USE / READING

☐ None ☐ Some ☐ A lot Total time: ______

☐ Sitting ☐ Standing ☐ Mixture Breaks every: ______

PHYSICAL ACTIVITY

☐ None ☐ Minimal ☐ Some ☐ Sweatin' ☐ I'm beat

DETAILS: ________________________________

RELIEF MEASURES

☐ Medication ☐ Massage ☐ Sleep ☐ Exercise

☐ Water ☐ Cold/Ice ☐ Heat/Bath ☐ Other

DETAILS: ________________________________

DID IT WORK? ☐ Nope ☐ A bit ☐ Mostly ☐ 100%

Notes

Entry #46

Date:________ M T W T F S S

START:		END:		DURATION:	

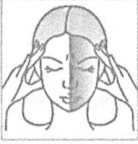

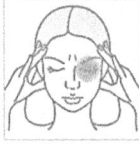

MIGRAINE CLUSTER SINUS TMJ TENSION

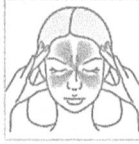

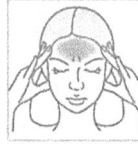

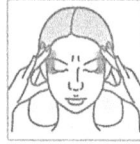

PAIN LEVEL

1	2	3	4	5	6	7	8	9	10

Not too bad. *Well, I'm not enjoying this.* *Make it stop!*

DETAILED DESCRIPTION

☐ Constant ☐ Squeezing ☐ Throbbing ☐ Pounding
☐ Dull aching ☐ Burning ☐ Sharp ☐ Debilitating

Other:______________________________

ONSET

☐ Slow ☐ Average ☐ Rapid ☐ Sudden

WHERE DOES IT HURT, EXACTLY?

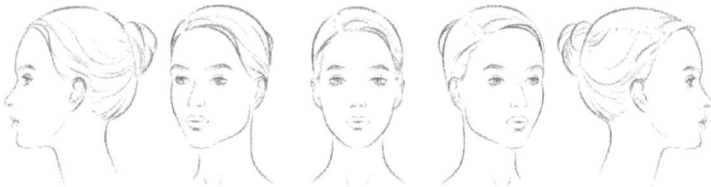

OTHER SYMPTOMS

☐ Lightheaded ☐ Dizziness ☐ Confusion
☐ Light sensitivity ☐ Sound sensitivity ☐ Auras
☐ Muscle stiffness ☐ Muscle burning ☐ Muscle aches

HOW ARE YOU FEELING OVERALL?

Mood	1	2	3	4	5	6	7	8	9	10
Energy levels	1	2	3	4	5	6	7	8	9	10
Mental clarity	1	2	3	4	5	6	7	8	9	10

Feeling sick?

☐ Nope!
☐ Yes...

☐ Nausea ☐ Diarrhea ☐ Vomiting ☐ Sore throat
☐ Congestion ☐ Coughing ☐ Chills ☐ Fever

Other symptoms: ______________________________

LAST NIGHT'S SLEEP

Hours of Sleep: ____________ Sleep Quality: ① ② ③ ④ ⑤

WEATHER

☐ Hot ☐ Mild ☐ Cold BM Pressure: ______
☐ Dry ☐ Humid ☐ Wet Allergen Levels: ______
☐ Sunny ☐ Cloudy

STRESS LEVELS

None	Low	Medium	High	Max	@$#%!

FOOD / DRINKS + NON-RELIEF MEDICATION / SUPPLEMENTS

item / meal	*time*	*meds / supplements*	*dose*	*time*

How many drinks?

water	→	1	2	3	4	5	6	7	8	9	10
caffeine	→	1	2	3	4	5	6	7	8	9	10
alcohol	→	1	2	3	4	5	6	7	8	9	10

HORMONES

☐ Menstruating ☐ Menopause ☐ PMS ☐ N/A | other

COMPUTER USE / READING

☐ None ☐ Some ☐ A lot Total time:
☐ Sitting ☐ Standing ☐ Mixture Breaks every:

PHYSICAL ACTIVITY

☐ None ☐ Minimal ☐ Some ☐ Sweatin' ☐ I'm beat

DETAILS: ____________

RELIEF MEASURES

☐ Medication ☐ Massage ☐ Sleep ☐ Exercise
☐ Water ☐ Cold/Ice ☐ Heat/Bath ☐ Other

DETAILS: ____________

DID IT WORK? ☐ Nope ☐ A bit ☐ Mostly ☐ 100%

Notes

Entry #47

Date:________ M T W T F S S

START:		END:		DURATION:	

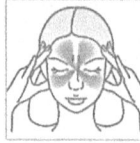

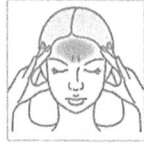

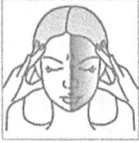

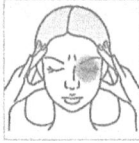

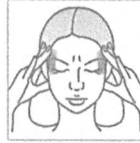

MIGRAINE CLUSTER SINUS TMJ TENSION

PAIN LEVEL

1	2	3	4	5	6	7	8	9	10

Not too bad. *Well, I'm not enjoying this.* *Make it stop!*

DETAILED DESCRIPTION

☐ Constant ☐ Squeezing ☐ Throbbing ☐ Pounding
☐ Dull aching ☐ Burning ☐ Sharp ☐ Debilitating

Other:____________________

ONSET

☐ Slow ☐ Average ☐ Rapid ☐ Sudden

WHERE DOES IT HURT, EXACTLY?

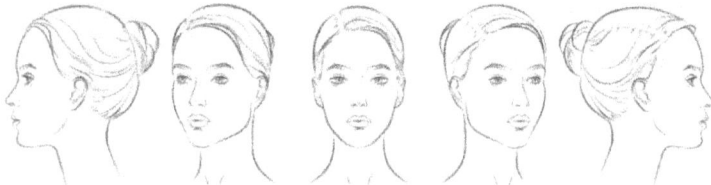

OTHER SYMPTOMS

☐ Lightheaded ☐ Dizziness ☐ Confusion
☐ Light sensitivity ☐ Sound sensitivity ☐ Auras
☐ Muscle stiffness ☐ Muscle burning ☐ Muscle aches

HOW ARE YOU FEELING OVERALL?

Mood	1	2	3	4	5	6	7	8	9	10
Energy levels	1	2	3	4	5	6	7	8	9	10
Mental clarity	1	2	3	4	5	6	7	8	9	10

Feeling sick?

☐ Nope!
☐ Yes...

☐ Nausea ☐ Diarrhea ☐ Vomiting ☐ Sore throat
☐ Congestion ☐ Coughing ☐ Chills ☐ Fever

Other symptoms: ____________________

LAST NIGHT'S SLEEP

Hours of Sleep: ______________ Sleep Quality: ① ② ③ ④ ⑤

WEATHER

☐ Hot ☐ Mild ☐ Cold BM Pressure: _______

☐ Dry ☐ Humid ☐ Wet Allergen Levels: _______

☐ Sunny ☐ Cloudy

STRESS LEVELS

None	Low	Medium	High	Max	@$#%!

FOOD / DRINKS + NON-RELIEF MEDICATION / SUPPLEMENTS

item / meal	*time*	*meds / supplements*	*dose*	*time*

How many drinks?

water	→	① ② ③ ④ ⑤ ⑥ ⑦ ⑧ ⑨ ⑩
caffeine	→	① ② ③ ④ ⑤ ⑥ ⑦ ⑧ ⑨ ⑩
alcohol	→	① ② ③ ④ ⑤ ⑥ ⑦ ⑧ ⑨ ⑩

HORMONES

☐ Menstruating ☐ Menopause ☐ PMS ☐ N/A | other

COMPUTER USE / READING

☐ None ☐ Some ☐ A lot Total time: ☐

☐ Sitting ☐ Standing ☐ Mixture Breaks every: ☐

PHYSICAL ACTIVITY

☐ None ☐ Minimal ☐ Some ☐ Sweatin' ☐ I'm beat

DETAILS: ______________________________

RELIEF MEASURES

☐ Medication ☐ Massage ☐ Sleep ☐ Exercise

☐ Water ☐ Cold/Ice ☐ Heat/Bath ☐ Other

DETAILS: ______________________________

DID IT WORK? ☐ Nope ☐ A bit ☐ Mostly ☐ 100%

Notes

Entry #48

Date:________ M T W T F S S

START:		END:		DURATION:	

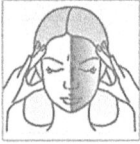

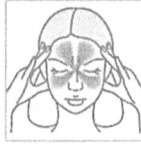

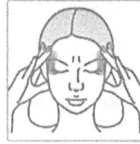

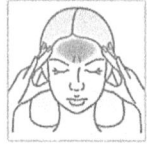

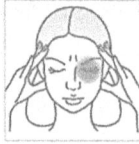

MIGRAINE CLUSTER SINUS TMJ TENSION

PAIN LEVEL

1	2	3	4	5	6	7	8	9	10

Not too bad. *Well, I'm not enjoying this.* *Make it stop!*

DETAILED DESCRIPTION

☐ Constant ☐ Squeezing ☐ Throbbing ☐ Pounding
☐ Dull aching ☐ Burning ☐ Sharp ☐ Debilitating

Other:______________________________

ONSET

☐ Slow ☐ Average ☐ Rapid ☐ Sudden

WHERE DOES IT HURT, EXACTLY?

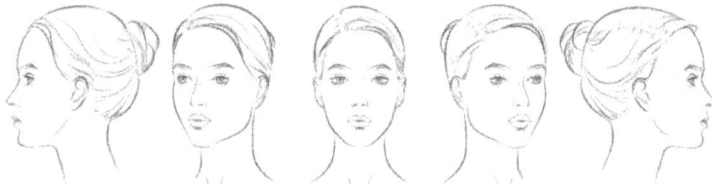

OTHER SYMPTOMS

☐ Lightheaded ☐ Dizziness ☐ Confusion
☐ Light sensitivity ☐ Sound sensitivity ☐ Auras
☐ Muscle stiffness ☐ Muscle burning ☐ Muscle aches

HOW ARE YOU FEELING OVERALL?

Mood	1	2	3	4	5	6	7	8	9	10
Energy levels	1	2	3	4	5	6	7	8	9	10
Mental clarity	1	2	3	4	5	6	7	8	9	10

Feeling sick?

☐ Nope!
☐ Yes...

☐ Nausea ☐ Diarrhea ☐ Vomiting ☐ Sore throat
☐ Congestion ☐ Coughing ☐ Chills ☐ Fever

Other symptoms:______________________________

LAST NIGHT'S SLEEP

Hours of Sleep: ____________ Sleep Quality: ① ② ③ ④ ⑤

WEATHER

☐ Hot ☐ Mild ☐ Cold BM Pressure: ______

☐ Dry ☐ Humid ☐ Wet Allergen Levels: ______

☐ Sunny ☐ Cloudy

STRESS LEVELS

None	Low	Medium	High	Max	@$#%!

FOOD / DRINKS + NON-RELIEF MEDICATION / SUPPLEMENTS

item / meal	*time*	*meds / supplements*	*dose*	*time*

How many drinks?

water	① ② ③ ④ ⑤ ⑥ ⑦ ⑧ ⑨ ⑩
caffeine	① ② ③ ④ ⑤ ⑥ ⑦ ⑧ ⑨ ⑩
alcohol	① ② ③ ④ ⑤ ⑥ ⑦ ⑧ ⑨ ⑩

HORMONES

☐ Menstruating ☐ Menopause ☐ PMS ☐ N/A | other

COMPUTER USE / READING

☐ None ☐ Some ☐ A lot Total time: ☐

☐ Sitting ☐ Standing ☐ Mixture Breaks every: ☐

PHYSICAL ACTIVITY

☐ None ☐ Minimal ☐ Some ☐ Sweatin' ☐ I'm beat

DETAILS: ________________________________

RELIEF MEASURES

☐ Medication ☐ Massage ☐ Sleep ☐ Exercise

☐ Water ☐ Cold/Ice ☐ Heat/Bath ☐ Other

DETAILS: ________________________________

DID IT WORK? ☐ Nope ☐ A bit ☐ Mostly ☐ 100%

Notes

Entry #49

Date:________ **M T W T F S S**

START:		END:		DURATION:	

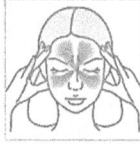

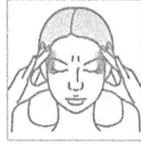

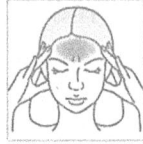

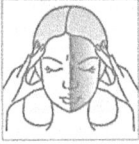

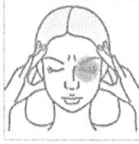

MIGRAINE CLUSTER SINUS TMJ TENSION

PAIN LEVEL

1	2	3	4	5	6	7	8	9	10

Not too bad. *Well, I'm not enjoying this.* *Make it stop!*

DETAILED DESCRIPTION

☐ Constant ☐ Squeezing ☐ Throbbing ☐ Pounding
☐ Dull aching ☐ Burning ☐ Sharp ☐ Debilitating

Other:____

ONSET

☐ Slow ☐ Average ☐ Rapid ☐ Sudden

WHERE DOES IT HURT, EXACTLY?

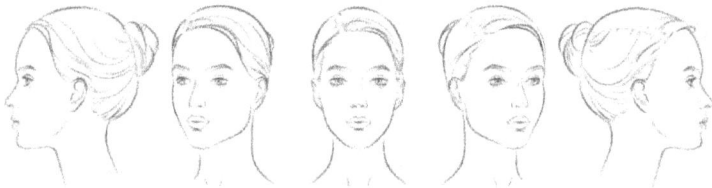

OTHER SYMPTOMS

☐ Lightheaded ☐ Dizziness ☐ Confusion
☐ Light sensitivity ☐ Sound sensitivity ☐ Auras
☐ Muscle stiffness ☐ Muscle burning ☐ Muscle aches

HOW ARE YOU FEELING OVERALL?

Mood	1	2	3	4	5	6	7	8	9	10
Energy levels	1	2	3	4	5	6	7	8	9	10
Mental clarity	1	2	3	4	5	6	7	8	9	10

Feeling sick?

☐ Nope!
☐ Yes...

☐ Nausea ☐ Diarrhea ☐ Vomiting ☐ Sore throat
☐ Congestion ☐ Coughing ☐ Chills ☐ Fever

Other symptoms: __________________________________

LAST NIGHT'S SLEEP

Hours of Sleep: ____________ Sleep Quality: (1) (2) (3) (4) (5)

WEATHER

☐ Hot ☐ Mild ☐ Cold BM Pressure: ______

☐ Dry ☐ Humid ☐ Wet Allergen Levels: ______

☐ Sunny ☐ Cloudy

STRESS LEVELS

None	Low	Medium	High	Max	@$#%!

FOOD / DRINKS + NON-RELIEF MEDICATION / SUPPLEMENTS

item / meal	*time*	*meds / supplements*	*dose*	*time*

How many drinks?

water →	(1)	(2)	(3)	(4)	(5)	(6)	(7)	(8)	(9)	(10)
caffeine →	(1)	(2)	(3)	(4)	(5)	(6)	(7)	(8)	(9)	(10)
alcohol →	(1)	(2)	(3)	(4)	(5)	(6)	(7)	(8)	(9)	(10)

HORMONES

☐ Menstruating ☐ Menopause ☐ PMS ☐ N/A | other

COMPUTER USE / READING

☐ None ☐ Some ☐ A lot Total time: ______

☐ Sitting ☐ Standing ☐ Mixture Breaks every: ______

PHYSICAL ACTIVITY

☐ None ☐ Minimal ☐ Some ☐ Sweatin' ☐ I'm beat

DETAILS: ________________________________

RELIEF MEASURES

☐ Medication ☐ Massage ☐ Sleep ☐ Exercise

☐ Water ☐ Cold/Ice ☐ Heat/Bath ☐ Other

DETAILS: ________________________________

DID IT WORK? ☐ Nope ☐ A bit ☐ Mostly ☐ 100%

Notes

Entry #50

Date:________ M T W T F S S

START:		END:		DURATION:	

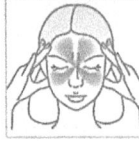

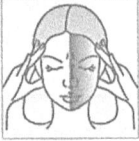

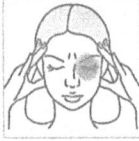

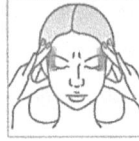

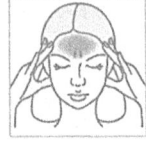

MIGRAINE CLUSTER SINUS TMJ TENSION

PAIN LEVEL

1	2	3	4	5	6	7	8	9	10

Not too bad. *Well, I'm not enjoying this.* *Make it stop!*

DETAILED DESCRIPTION

☐ Constant ☐ Squeezing ☐ Throbbing ☐ Pounding
☐ Dull aching ☐ Burning ☐ Sharp ☐ Debilitating

Other:________________

ONSET

☐ Slow ☐ Average ☐ Rapid ☐ Sudden

WHERE DOES IT HURT, EXACTLY?

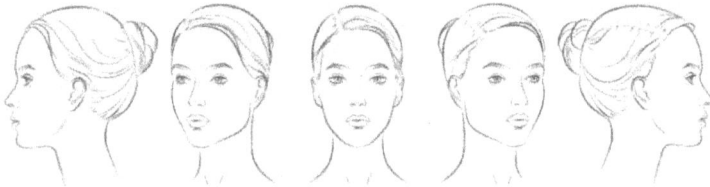

OTHER SYMPTOMS

☐ Lightheaded ☐ Dizziness ☐ Confusion
☐ Light sensitivity ☐ Sound sensitivity ☐ Auras
☐ Muscle stiffness ☐ Muscle burning ☐ Muscle aches

HOW ARE YOU FEELING OVERALL?

Mood	1	2	3	4	5	6	7	8	9	10
Energy levels	1	2	3	4	5	6	7	8	9	10
Mental clarity	1	2	3	4	5	6	7	8	9	10

Feeling sick?

☐ Nope!
☐ Yes...

☐ Nausea ☐ Diarrhea ☐ Vomiting ☐ Sore throat
☐ Congestion ☐ Coughing ☐ Chills ☐ Fever

Other symptoms: ________________

LAST NIGHT'S SLEEP

Hours of Sleep: ____________ Sleep Quality: ① ② ③ ④ ⑤

WEATHER

☐ Hot ☐ Mild ☐ Cold BM Pressure: ______

☐ Dry ☐ Humid ☐ Wet Allergen Levels: ______

☐ Sunny ☐ Cloudy

STRESS LEVELS

None	Low	Medium	High	Max	@$#%!

FOOD / DRINKS + NON-RELIEF MEDICATION / SUPPLEMENTS

item / meal	*time*	*meds / supplements*	*dose*	*time*

How many drinks?

water	① ② ③ ④ ⑤ ⑥ ⑦ ⑧ ⑨ ⑩
caffeine	① ② ③ ④ ⑤ ⑥ ⑦ ⑧ ⑨ ⑩
alcohol	① ② ③ ④ ⑤ ⑥ ⑦ ⑧ ⑨ ⑩

HORMONES

☐ Menstruating ☐ Menopause ☐ PMS ☐ N/A | other

COMPUTER USE / READING

☐ None ☐ Some ☐ A lot Total time:

☐ Sitting ☐ Standing ☐ Mixture Breaks every:

PHYSICAL ACTIVITY

☐ None ☐ Minimal ☐ Some ☐ Sweatin' ☐ I'm beat

DETAILS: ____________________

RELIEF MEASURES

☐ Medication ☐ Massage ☐ Sleep ☐ Exercise

☐ Water ☐ Cold/Ice ☐ Heat/Bath ☐ Other

DETAILS: ____________________

DID IT WORK? ☐ Nope ☐ A bit ☐ Mostly ☐ 100%

Notes

Entry #51

Date:________ M T W T F S S

START:		END:		DURATION:	

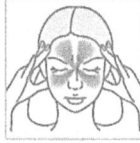

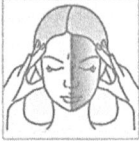

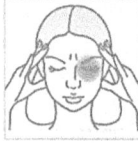

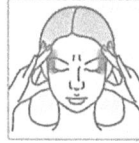

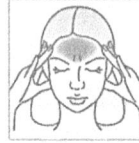

MIGRAINE CLUSTER SINUS TMJ TENSION

PAIN LEVEL

1	2	3	4	5	6	7	8	9	10

Not too bad. *Well, I'm not enjoying this.* *Make it stop!*

DETAILED DESCRIPTION

☐ Constant ☐ Squeezing ☐ Throbbing ☐ Pounding
☐ Dull aching ☐ Burning ☐ Sharp ☐ Debilitating

Other:________________________________

ONSET

☐ Slow ☐ Average ☐ Rapid ☐ Sudden

WHERE DOES IT HURT, EXACTLY?

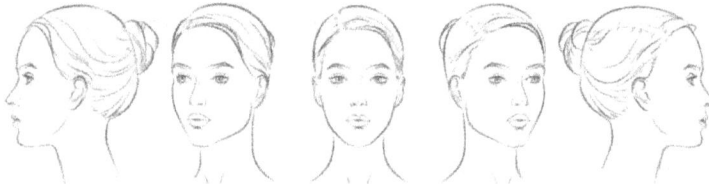

OTHER SYMPTOMS

☐ Lightheaded ☐ Dizziness ☐ Confusion
☐ Light sensitivity ☐ Sound sensitivity ☐ Auras
☐ Muscle stiffness ☐ Muscle burning ☐ Muscle aches

HOW ARE YOU FEELING OVERALL?

		Feeling sick?
Mood	① ② ③ ④ ⑤ ⑥ ⑦ ⑧ ⑨ ⑩	☐ Nope!
Energy levels	① ② ③ ④ ⑤ ⑥ ⑦ ⑧ ⑨ ⑩	☐ Yes...
Mental clarity	① ② ③ ④ ⑤ ⑥ ⑦ ⑧ ⑨ ⑩	

☐ Nausea ☐ Diarrhea ☐ Vomiting ☐ Sore throat
☐ Congestion ☐ Coughing ☐ Chills ☐ Fever

Other symptoms: ______________________________

LAST NIGHT'S SLEEP

Hours of Sleep: ____________ Sleep Quality: ① ② ③ ④ ⑤

WEATHER

☐ Hot ☐ Mild ☐ Cold BM Pressure: ______

☐ Dry ☐ Humid ☐ Wet Allergen Levels: ______

☐ Sunny ☐ Cloudy

STRESS LEVELS

None	Low	Medium	High	Max	@$#%!

FOOD / DRINKS + NON-RELIEF MEDICATION / SUPPLEMENTS

item / meal	*time*	*meds / supplements*	*dose*	*time*

How many drinks?

water	1	2	3	4	5	6	7	8	9	10
caffeine	1	2	3	4	5	6	7	8	9	10
alcohol	1	2	3	4	5	6	7	8	9	10

HORMONES

☐ Menstruating ☐ Menopause ☐ PMS ☐ N/A | other

COMPUTER USE / READING

☐ None ☐ Some ☐ A lot Total time: ______

☐ Sitting ☐ Standing ☐ Mixture Breaks every: ______

PHYSICAL ACTIVITY

☐ None ☐ Minimal ☐ Some ☐ Sweatin' ☐ I'm beat

DETAILS: ____

RELIEF MEASURES

☐ Medication ☐ Massage ☐ Sleep ☐ Exercise

☐ Water ☐ Cold/Ice ☐ Heat/Bath ☐ Other

DETAILS: ____

DID IT WORK? ☐ Nope ☐ A bit ☐ Mostly ☐ 100%

Notes

Entry #52

Date:________ M T W T F S S

START:		END:		DURATION:	

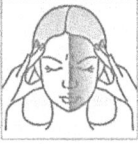

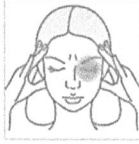

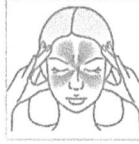

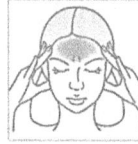

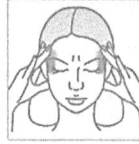

MIGRAINE CLUSTER SINUS TMJ TENSION

PAIN LEVEL

1	2	3	4	5	6	7	8	9	10

Not too bad. *Well, I'm not enjoying this.* *Make it stop!*

DETAILED DESCRIPTION

☐ Constant ☐ Squeezing ☐ Throbbing ☐ Pounding
☐ Dull aching ☐ Burning ☐ Sharp ☐ Debilitating

Other:____________________

ONSET

☐ Slow ☐ Average ☐ Rapid ☐ Sudden

WHERE DOES IT HURT, EXACTLY?

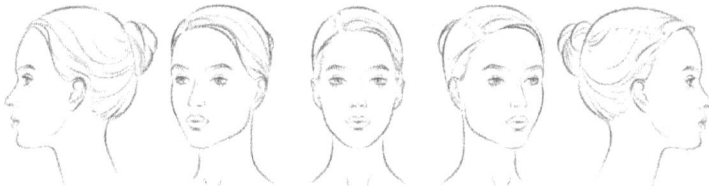

OTHER SYMPTOMS

☐ Lightheaded ☐ Dizziness ☐ Confusion
☐ Light sensitivity ☐ Sound sensitivity ☐ Auras
☐ Muscle stiffness ☐ Muscle burning ☐ Muscle aches

HOW ARE YOU FEELING OVERALL?

Mood	1	2	3	4	5	6	7	8	9	10
Energy levels	1	2	3	4	5	6	7	8	9	10
Mental clarity	1	2	3	4	5	6	7	8	9	10

Feeling sick?

☐ Nope!
☐ Yes...

☐ Nausea ☐ Diarrhea ☐ Vomiting ☐ Sore throat
☐ Congestion ☐ Coughing ☐ Chills ☐ Fever

Other symptoms: ____________________

LAST NIGHT'S SLEEP

Hours of Sleep: ______________ Sleep Quality: ① ② ③ ④ ⑤

WEATHER

☐ Hot ☐ Mild ☐ Cold BM Pressure: _______

☐ Dry ☐ Humid ☐ Wet Allergen Levels: _______

☐ Sunny ☐ Cloudy

STRESS LEVELS

None	Low	Medium	High	Max	@$#%!

FOOD / DRINKS + NON-RELIEF MEDICATION / SUPPLEMENTS

item / meal	*time*	*meds / supplements*	*dose*	*time*

How many drinks?

water	① ② ③ ④ ⑤ ⑥ ⑦ ⑧ ⑨ ⑩
caffeine	① ② ③ ④ ⑤ ⑥ ⑦ ⑧ ⑨ ⑩
alcohol	① ② ③ ④ ⑤ ⑥ ⑦ ⑧ ⑨ ⑩

HORMONES

☐ Menstruating ☐ Menopause ☐ PMS ☐ N/A | other

COMPUTER USE / READING

☐ None ☐ Some ☐ A lot Total time:

☐ Sitting ☐ Standing ☐ Mixture Breaks every:

PHYSICAL ACTIVITY

☐ None ☐ Minimal ☐ Some ☐ Sweatin' ☐ I'm beat

DETAILS: ____

RELIEF MEASURES

☐ Medication ☐ Massage ☐ Sleep ☐ Exercise

☐ Water ☐ Cold/Ice ☐ Heat/Bath ☐ Other

DETAILS: ____

DID IT WORK? ☐ Nope ☐ A bit ☐ Mostly ☐ 100%

Notes

Entry #53

Date:_______ **M T W T F S S**

START:		END:		DURATION:	

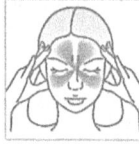

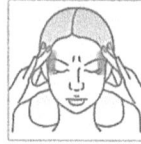

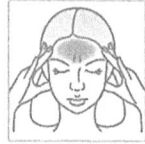

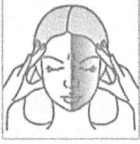

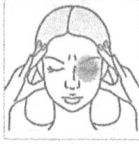

MIGRAINE CLUSTER SINUS TMJ TENSION

PAIN LEVEL

1	2	3	4	5	6	7	8	9	10

Not too bad. *Well, I'm not enjoying this.* *Make it stop!*

DETAILED DESCRIPTION

☐ Constant ☐ Squeezing ☐ Throbbing ☐ Pounding
☐ Dull aching ☐ Burning ☐ Sharp ☐ Debilitating

Other:________________________________

ONSET

☐ Slow ☐ Average ☐ Rapid ☐ Sudden

WHERE DOES IT HURT, EXACTLY?

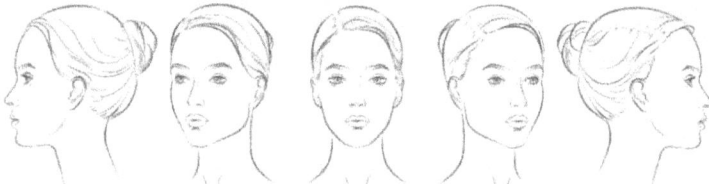

OTHER SYMPTOMS

☐ Lightheaded ☐ Dizziness ☐ Confusion
☐ Light sensitivity ☐ Sound sensitivity ☐ Auras
☐ Muscle stiffness ☐ Muscle burning ☐ Muscle aches

HOW ARE YOU FEELING OVERALL?

Mood	1	2	3	4	5	6	7	8	9	10
Energy levels	1	2	3	4	5	6	7	8	9	10
Mental clarity	1	2	3	4	5	6	7	8	9	10

Feeling sick?

☐ Nope!
☐ Yes...

☐ Nausea ☐ Diarrhea ☐ Vomiting ☐ Sore throat
☐ Congestion ☐ Coughing ☐ Chills ☐ Fever

Other symptoms: ________________________

LAST NIGHT'S SLEEP

Hours of Sleep: ____________ Sleep Quality: ① ② ③ ④ ⑤

WEATHER

☐ Hot ☐ Mild ☐ Cold BM Pressure: ______

☐ Dry ☐ Humid ☐ Wet Allergen Levels: ______

☐ Sunny ☐ Cloudy

STRESS LEVELS

None	Low	Medium	High	Max	@$#%!

FOOD / DRINKS + NON-RELIEF MEDICATION / SUPPLEMENTS

item / meal	*time*	*meds / supplements*	*dose*	*time*

How many drinks?

water	① ② ③ ④ ⑤ ⑥ ⑦ ⑧ ⑨ ⑩
caffeine	① ② ③ ④ ⑤ ⑥ ⑦ ⑧ ⑨ ⑩
alcohol	① ② ③ ④ ⑤ ⑥ ⑦ ⑧ ⑨ ⑩

HORMONES

☐ Menstruating ☐ Menopause ☐ PMS ☐ N/A | other

COMPUTER USE / READING

☐ None ☐ Some ☐ A lot Total time: ______

☐ Sitting ☐ Standing ☐ Mixture Breaks every: ______

PHYSICAL ACTIVITY

☐ None ☐ Minimal ☐ Some ☐ Sweatin' ☐ I'm beat

DETAILS: ____

RELIEF MEASURES

☐ Medication ☐ Massage ☐ Sleep ☐ Exercise

☐ Water ☐ Cold/Ice ☐ Heat/Bath ☐ Other

DETAILS: ____

DID IT WORK? ☐ Nope ☐ A bit ☐ Mostly ☐ 100%

Notes

Entry #54

Date:________ **M T W T F S S**

START: ______ END: ______ DURATION: ______

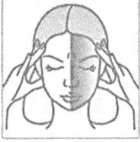

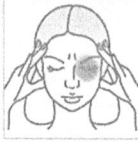

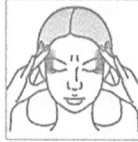

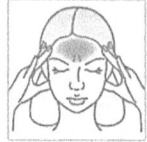

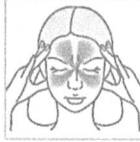

MIGRAINE CLUSTER SINUS TMJ TENSION

PAIN LEVEL

1	2	3	4	5	6	7	8	9	10

Not too bad. *Well, I'm not enjoying this.* *Make it stop!*

DETAILED DESCRIPTION

☐ Constant ☐ Squeezing ☐ Throbbing ☐ Pounding
☐ Dull aching ☐ Burning ☐ Sharp ☐ Debilitating

Other:________________________________

ONSET

☐ Slow ☐ Average ☐ Rapid ☐ Sudden

WHERE DOES IT HURT, EXACTLY?

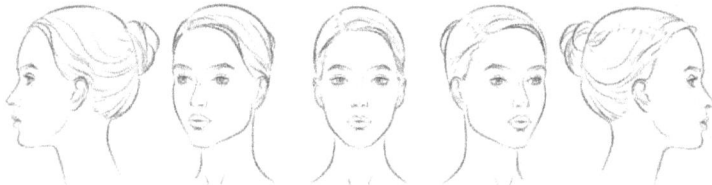

OTHER SYMPTOMS

☐ Lightheaded ☐ Dizziness ☐ Confusion
☐ Light sensitivity ☐ Sound sensitivity ☐ Auras
☐ Muscle stiffness ☐ Muscle burning ☐ Muscle aches

HOW ARE YOU FEELING OVERALL?

Mood	1	2	3	4	5	6	7	8	9	10
Energy levels	1	2	3	4	5	6	7	8	9	10
Mental clarity	1	2	3	4	5	6	7	8	9	10

Feeling sick?

☐ Nope!
☐ Yes...

☐ Nausea ☐ Diarrhea ☐ Vomiting ☐ Sore throat
☐ Congestion ☐ Coughing ☐ Chills ☐ Fever

Other symptoms: ________________________________

LAST NIGHT'S SLEEP

Hours of Sleep: ____________ Sleep Quality: ① ② ③ ④ ⑤

WEATHER

☐ Hot ☐ Mild ☐ Cold BM Pressure: ______

☐ Dry ☐ Humid ☐ Wet Allergen Levels: ______

☐ Sunny ☐ Cloudy

STRESS LEVELS

None	Low	Medium	High	Max	@$#%!

FOOD / DRINKS + NON-RELIEF MEDICATION / SUPPLEMENTS

item / meal	*time*	*meds / supplements*	*dose*	*time*

How many drinks?

water	① ② ③ ④ ⑤ ⑥ ⑦ ⑧ ⑨ ⑩
caffeine	① ② ③ ④ ⑤ ⑥ ⑦ ⑧ ⑨ ⑩
alcohol	① ② ③ ④ ⑤ ⑥ ⑦ ⑧ ⑨ ⑩

HORMONES

☐ Menstruating ☐ Menopause ☐ PMS ☐ N/A | other

COMPUTER USE / READING

☐ None ☐ Some ☐ A lot Total time: ______

☐ Sitting ☐ Standing ☐ Mixture Breaks every: ______

PHYSICAL ACTIVITY

☐ None ☐ Minimal ☐ Some ☐ Sweatin' ☐ I'm beat

DETAILS: ______________________________

RELIEF MEASURES

☐ Medication ☐ Massage ☐ Sleep ☐ Exercise

☐ Water ☐ Cold/Ice ☐ Heat/Bath ☐ Other

DETAILS: ______________________________

DID IT WORK? ☐ Nope ☐ A bit ☐ Mostly ☐ 100%

Notes

Entry #55

Date:________ M T W T F S S

START: | END: | DURATION:

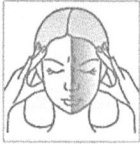

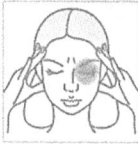

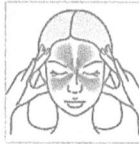

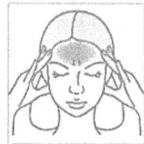

MIGRAINE CLUSTER SINUS TMJ TENSION

PAIN LEVEL

1	2	3	4	5	6	7	8	9	10

Not too bad. *Well, I'm not enjoying this.* *Make it stop!*

DETAILED DESCRIPTION

☐ Constant ☐ Squeezing ☐ Throbbing ☐ Pounding
☐ Dull aching ☐ Burning ☐ Sharp ☐ Debilitating

Other:____________________

ONSET

☐ Slow ☐ Average ☐ Rapid ☐ Sudden

WHERE DOES IT HURT, EXACTLY?

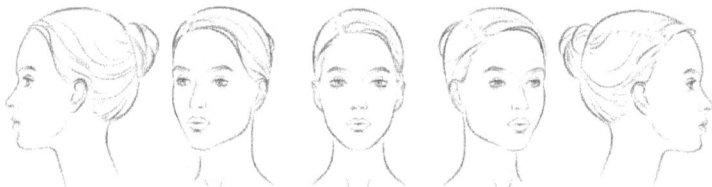

OTHER SYMPTOMS

☐ Lightheaded ☐ Dizziness ☐ Confusion
☐ Light sensitivity ☐ Sound sensitivity ☐ Auras
☐ Muscle stiffness ☐ Muscle burning ☐ Muscle aches

HOW ARE YOU FEELING OVERALL?

Mood	1	2	3	4	5	6	7	8	9	10
Energy levels	1	2	3	4	5	6	7	8	9	10
Mental clarity	1	2	3	4	5	6	7	8	9	10

Feeling sick?

☐ Nope!
☐ Yes...

☐ Nausea ☐ Diarrhea ☐ Vomiting ☐ Sore throat
☐ Congestion ☐ Coughing ☐ Chills ☐ Fever

Other symptoms: ____________________

LAST NIGHT'S SLEEP

Hours of Sleep: ____________ Sleep Quality: ① ② ③ ④ ⑤

WEATHER

☐ Hot ☐ Mild ☐ Cold BM Pressure: ______

☐ Dry ☐ Humid ☐ Wet Allergen Levels: ______

☐ Sunny ☐ Cloudy

STRESS LEVELS

None	Low	Medium	High	Max	@$#%!

FOOD / DRINKS + NON-RELIEF MEDICATION / SUPPLEMENTS

item / meal	*time*	*meds / supplements*	*dose*	*time*

How many drinks?

water	① ② ③ ④ ⑤ ⑥ ⑦ ⑧ ⑨ ⑩
caffeine	① ② ③ ④ ⑤ ⑥ ⑦ ⑧ ⑨ ⑩
alcohol	① ② ③ ④ ⑤ ⑥ ⑦ ⑧ ⑨ ⑩

HORMONES

☐ Menstruating ☐ Menopause ☐ PMS ☐ N/A | other

COMPUTER USE / READING

☐ None ☐ Some ☐ A lot Total time:

☐ Sitting ☐ Standing ☐ Mixture Breaks every:

PHYSICAL ACTIVITY

☐ None ☐ Minimal ☐ Some ☐ Sweatin' ☐ I'm beat

DETAILS: ________________________________

RELIEF MEASURES

☐ Medication ☐ Massage ☐ Sleep ☐ Exercise

☐ Water ☐ Cold/Ice ☐ Heat/Bath ☐ Other

DETAILS: ________________________________

DID IT WORK? ☐ Nope ☐ A bit ☐ Mostly ☐ 100%

Notes

Entry #56

Date:________ M T W T F S S

START:		END:		DURATION:	

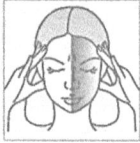

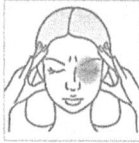

MIGRAINE CLUSTER SINUS TMJ TENSION

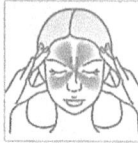

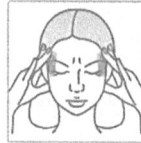

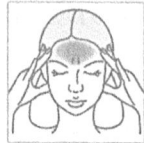

PAIN LEVEL

1	2	3	4	5	6	7	8	9	10

Not too bad. *Well, I'm not enjoying this.* *Make it stop!*

DETAILED DESCRIPTION

☐ Constant ☐ Squeezing ☐ Throbbing ☐ Pounding
☐ Dull aching ☐ Burning ☐ Sharp ☐ Debilitating

Other:____________________

ONSET

☐ Slow ☐ Average ☐ Rapid ☐ Sudden

WHERE DOES IT HURT, EXACTLY?

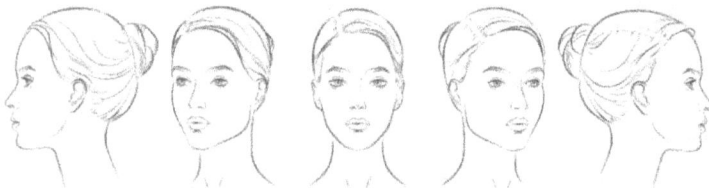

OTHER SYMPTOMS

☐ Lightheaded ☐ Dizziness ☐ Confusion
☐ Light sensitivity ☐ Sound sensitivity ☐ Auras
☐ Muscle stiffness ☐ Muscle burning ☐ Muscle aches

HOW AREA YOU FEELING OVERALL?

		Feeling sick?
Mood	① ② ③ ④ ⑤ ⑥ ⑦ ⑧ ⑨ ⑩	☐ Nope!
Energy levels	① ② ③ ④ ⑤ ⑥ ⑦ ⑧ ⑨ ⑩	☐ Yes...
Mental clarity	① ② ③ ④ ⑤ ⑥ ⑦ ⑧ ⑨ ⑩	

☐ Nausea ☐ Diarrhea ☐ Vomiting ☐ Sore throat
☐ Congestion ☐ Coughing ☐ Chills ☐ Fever

Other symptoms:____________________

LAST NIGHT'S SLEEP

Hours of Sleep: ____________ Sleep Quality: ① ② ③ ④ ⑤

WEATHER

☐ Hot ☐ Mild ☐ Cold BM Pressure: ______

☐ Dry ☐ Humid ☐ Wet Allergen Levels: ______

☐ Sunny ☐ Cloudy

STRESS LEVELS

None	Low	Medium	High	Max	@$#%!

FOOD / DRINKS + NON-RELIEF MEDICATION / SUPPLEMENTS

item / meal	*time*	*meds / supplements*	*dose*	*time*

How many drinks?

water	① ② ③ ④ ⑤ ⑥ ⑦ ⑧ ⑨ ⑩
caffeine	① ② ③ ④ ⑤ ⑥ ⑦ ⑧ ⑨ ⑩
alcohol	① ② ③ ④ ⑤ ⑥ ⑦ ⑧ ⑨ ⑩

HORMONES

☐ Menstruating ☐ Menopause ☐ PMS ☐ N/A | other

COMPUTER USE / READING

☐ None ☐ Some ☐ A lot Total time:

☐ Sitting ☐ Standing ☐ Mixture Breaks every:

PHYSICAL ACTIVITY

☐ None ☐ Minimal ☐ Some ☐ Sweatin' ☐ I'm beat

DETAILS: ______________________________

RELIEF MEASURES

☐ Medication ☐ Massage ☐ Sleep ☐ Exercise

☐ Water ☐ Cold/Ice ☐ Heat/Bath ☐ Other

DETAILS: ______________________________

DID IT WORK? ☐ Nope ☐ A bit ☐ Mostly ☐ 100%

Notes

Entry #57

Date:________ M T W T F S S

START:		END:		DURATION:	

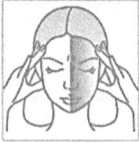

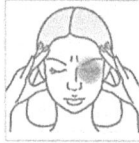

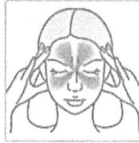

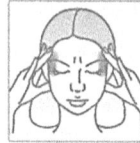

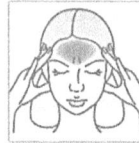

MIGRAINE CLUSTER SINUS TMJ TENSION

PAIN LEVEL

1	2	3	4	5	6	7	8	9	10

Not too bad. *Well, I'm not enjoying this.* *Make it stop!*

DETAILED DESCRIPTION

☐ Constant ☐ Squeezing ☐ Throbbing ☐ Pounding
☐ Dull aching ☐ Burning ☐ Sharp ☐ Debilitating

Other:____

ONSET

☐ Slow ☐ Average ☐ Rapid ☐ Sudden

WHERE DOES IT HURT, EXACTLY?

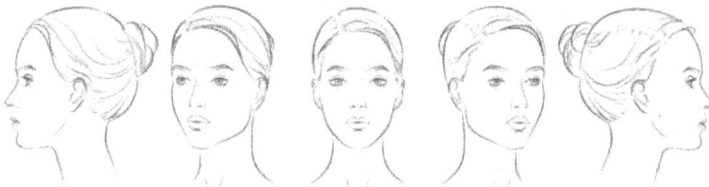

OTHER SYMPTOMS

☐ Lightheaded ☐ Dizziness ☐ Confusion
☐ Light sensitivity ☐ Sound sensitivity ☐ Auras
☐ Muscle stiffness ☐ Muscle burning ☐ Muscle aches

HOW ARE YOU FEELING OVERALL?

		Feeling sick?
Mood	① ② ③ ④ ⑤ ⑥ ⑦ ⑧ ⑨ ⑩	☐ Nope!
Energy levels	① ② ③ ④ ⑤ ⑥ ⑦ ⑧ ⑨ ⑩	☐ Yes...
Mental clarity	① ② ③ ④ ⑤ ⑥ ⑦ ⑧ ⑨ ⑩	

☐ Nausea ☐ Diarrhea ☐ Vomiting ☐ Sore throat
☐ Congestion ☐ Coughing ☐ Chills ☐ Fever

Other symptoms: ________________________________

LAST NIGHT'S SLEEP

Hours of Sleep: ____________ Sleep Quality: ① ② ③ ④ ⑤

WEATHER

☐ Hot ☐ Mild ☐ Cold BM Pressure: ______

☐ Dry ☐ Humid ☐ Wet Allergen Levels: ______

☐ Sunny ☐ Cloudy

STRESS LEVELS

None	Low	Medium	High	Max	@$#%!

FOOD / DRINKS + NON-RELIEF MEDICATION / SUPPLEMENTS

item / meal	*time*	*meds / supplements*	*dose*	*time*
		How many drinks?		

water	→	① ② ③ ④ ⑤ ⑥ ⑦ ⑧ ⑨ ⑩
caffeine	→	① ② ③ ④ ⑤ ⑥ ⑦ ⑧ ⑨ ⑩
alcohol	→	① ② ③ ④ ⑤ ⑥ ⑦ ⑧ ⑨ ⑩

HORMONES

☐ Menstruating ☐ Menopause ☐ PMS ☐ N/A | other

COMPUTER USE / READING

☐ None ☐ Some ☐ A lot Total time: ☐

☐ Sitting ☐ Standing ☐ Mixture Breaks every: ☐

PHYSICAL ACTIVITY

☐ None ☐ Minimal ☐ Some ☐ Sweatin' ☐ I'm beat

DETAILS: ______________________________

RELIEF MEASURES

☐ Medication ☐ Massage ☐ Sleep ☐ Exercise

☐ Water ☐ Cold/Ice ☐ Heat/Bath ☐ Other

DETAILS: ______________________________

DID IT WORK? ☐ Nope ☐ A bit ☐ Mostly ☐ 100%

Notes

Entry #58

Date:________ M T W T F S S

START:		END:		DURATION:	

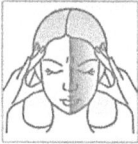

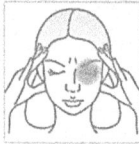

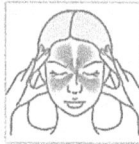

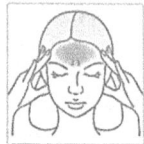

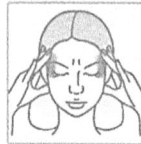

MIGRAINE CLUSTER SINUS TMJ TENSION

PAIN LEVEL

1	2	3	4	5	6	7	8	9	10

Not too bad. *Well, I'm not enjoying this.* *Make it stop!*

DETAILED DESCRIPTION

☐ Constant ☐ Squeezing ☐ Throbbing ☐ Pounding
☐ Dull aching ☐ Burning ☐ Sharp ☐ Debilitating

Other:______________________________

ONSET

☐ Slow ☐ Average ☐ Rapid ☐ Sudden

WHERE DOES IT HURT, EXACTLY?

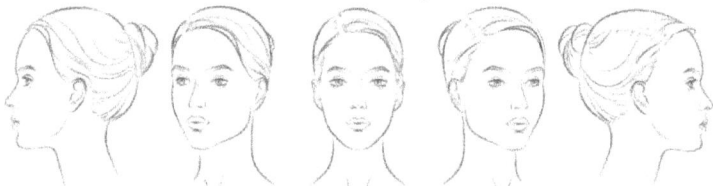

OTHER SYMPTOMS

☐ Lightheaded ☐ Dizziness ☐ Confusion
☐ Light sensitivity ☐ Sound sensitivity ☐ Auras
☐ Muscle stiffness ☐ Muscle burning ☐ Muscle aches

HOW ARE YOU FEELING OVERALL?

Mood	1	2	3	4	5	6	7	8	9	10
Energy levels	1	2	3	4	5	6	7	8	9	10
Mental clarity	1	2	3	4	5	6	7	8	9	10

Feeling sick?

☐ Nope!
☐ Yes...

☐ Nausea ☐ Diarrhea ☐ Vomiting ☐ Sore throat
☐ Congestion ☐ Coughing ☐ Chills ☐ Fever

Other symptoms: ______________________________

LAST NIGHT'S SLEEP

Hours of Sleep: ____________ Sleep Quality: ① ② ③ ④ ⑤

WEATHER

☐ Hot ☐ Mild ☐ Cold BM Pressure: ______
☐ Dry ☐ Humid ☐ Wet Allergen Levels: ______
☐ Sunny ☐ Cloudy

STRESS LEVELS

None	Low	Medium	High	Max	@$#%!

FOOD / DRINKS + NON-RELIEF MEDICATION / SUPPLEMENTS

item / meal	*time*	*meds / supplements*	*dose*	*time*
		How many drinks?		

water	→	① ② ③ ④ ⑤ ⑥ ⑦ ⑧ ⑨ ⑩
caffeine	→	① ② ③ ④ ⑤ ⑥ ⑦ ⑧ ⑨ ⑩
alcohol	→	① ② ③ ④ ⑤ ⑥ ⑦ ⑧ ⑨ ⑩

HORMONES

☐ Menstruating ☐ Menopause ☐ PMS ☐ N/A | other

COMPUTER USE / READING

☐ None ☐ Some ☐ A lot Total time: ______
☐ Sitting ☐ Standing ☐ Mixture Breaks every: ______

PHYSICAL ACTIVITY

☐ None ☐ Minimal ☐ Some ☐ Sweatin' ☐ I'm beat

DETAILS: ____

RELIEF MEASURES

☐ Medication ☐ Massage ☐ Sleep ☐ Exercise
☐ Water ☐ Cold/Ice ☐ Heat/Bath ☐ Other

DETAILS: ____

DID IT WORK? ☐ Nope ☐ A bit ☐ Mostly ☐ 100%

Notes

Entry #59

Date:_______ M T W T F S S

START:		END:		DURATION:	

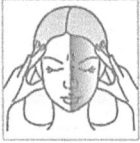

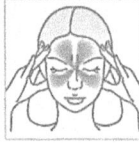

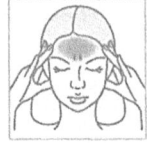

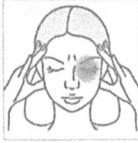

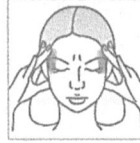

MIGRAINE CLUSTER SINUS TMJ TENSION

PAIN LEVEL

1	2	3	4	5	6	7	8	9	10

Not too bad. *Well, I'm not enjoying this.* *Make it stop!*

DETAILED DESCRIPTION

☐ Constant ☐ Squeezing ☐ Throbbing ☐ Pounding
☐ Dull aching ☐ Burning ☐ Sharp ☐ Debilitating

Other:________________________________

ONSET

☐ Slow ☐ Average ☐ Rapid ☐ Sudden

WHERE DOES IT HURT, EXACTLY?

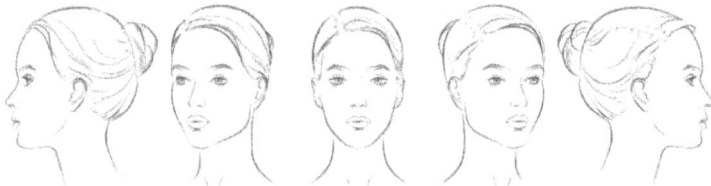

OTHER SYMPTOMS

☐ Lightheaded ☐ Dizziness ☐ Confusion
☐ Light sensitivity ☐ Sound sensitivity ☐ Auras
☐ Muscle stiffness ☐ Muscle burning ☐ Muscle aches

HOW ARE YOU FEELING OVERALL?

Mood	1	2	3	4	5	6	7	8	9	10
Energy levels	1	2	3	4	5	6	7	8	9	10
Mental clarity	1	2	3	4	5	6	7	8	9	10

Feeling sick?

☐ Nope!
☐ Yes...

☐ Nausea ☐ Diarrhea ☐ Vomiting ☐ Sore throat
☐ Congestion ☐ Coughing ☐ Chills ☐ Fever

Other symptoms: ________________________________

LAST NIGHT'S SLEEP

Hours of Sleep: ____________ Sleep Quality: (1) (2) (3) (4) (5)

WEATHER

☐ Hot ☐ Mild ☐ Cold BM Pressure: ______

☐ Dry ☐ Humid ☐ Wet Allergen Levels: ______

☐ Sunny ☐ Cloudy

STRESS LEVELS

None	Low	Medium	High	Max	@$#%!

FOOD / DRINKS + NON-RELIEF MEDICATION / SUPPLEMENTS

item / meal	*time*	*meds / supplements*	*dose*	*time*
		How many drinks?		

		How many drinks?
water	⇨	(1) (2) (3) (4) (5) (6) (7) (8) (9) (10)
caffeine	⇨	(1) (2) (3) (4) (5) (6) (7) (8) (9) (10)
alcohol	⇨	(1) (2) (3) (4) (5) (6) (7) (8) (9) (10)

HORMONES

☐ Menstruating ☐ Menopause ☐ PMS ☐ N/A | other

COMPUTER USE / READING

☐ None ☐ Some ☐ A lot Total time: ______

☐ Sitting ☐ Standing ☐ Mixture Breaks every: ______

PHYSICAL ACTIVITY

☐ None ☐ Minimal ☐ Some ☐ Sweatin' ☐ I'm beat

DETAILS: ______________________________

RELIEF MEASURES

☐ Medication ☐ Massage ☐ Sleep ☐ Exercise

☐ Water ☐ Cold/Ice ☐ Heat/Bath ☐ Other

DETAILS: ______________________________

DID IT WORK? ☐ Nope ☐ A bit ☐ Mostly ☐ 100%

Notes

Entry #60

Date:________ M T W T F S S

START:		END:		DURATION:	

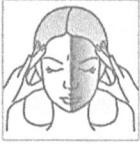

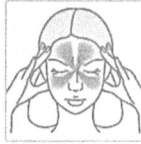

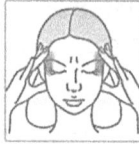

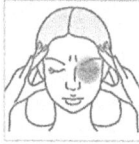

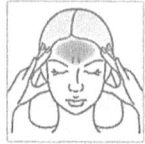

MIGRAINE CLUSTER SINUS TMJ TENSION

PAIN LEVEL

1	2	3	4	5	6	7	8	9	10

Not too bad. *Well, I'm not enjoying this.* *Make it stop!*

DETAILED DESCRIPTION

- ☐ Constant ☐ Squeezing ☐ Throbbing ☐ Pounding
- ☐ Dull aching ☐ Burning ☐ Sharp ☐ Debilitating

Other:____________________

ONSET

☐ Slow ☐ Average ☐ Rapid ☐ Sudden

WHERE DOES IT HURT, EXACTLY?

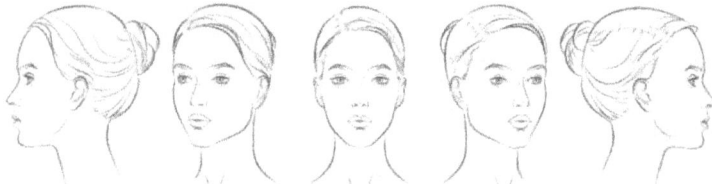

OTHER SYMPTOMS

- ☐ Lightheaded ☐ Dizziness ☐ Confusion
- ☐ Light sensitivity ☐ Sound sensitivity ☐ Auras
- ☐ Muscle stiffness ☐ Muscle burning ☐ Muscle aches

HOW ARE YOU FEELING OVERALL?

Mood	① ② ③ ④ ⑤ ⑥ ⑦ ⑧ ⑨ ⑩	☐ Nope!
Energy levels	① ② ③ ④ ⑤ ⑥ ⑦ ⑧ ⑨ ⑩	☐ Yes...
Mental clarity	① ② ③ ④ ⑤ ⑥ ⑦ ⑧ ⑨ ⑩	

Feeling sick?

- ☐ Nausea ☐ Diarrhea ☐ Vomiting ☐ Sore throat
- ☐ Congestion ☐ Coughing ☐ Chills ☐ Fever

Other symptoms: ____________________

LAST NIGHT'S SLEEP

Hours of Sleep: ____________ Sleep Quality: ① ② ③ ④ ⑤

WEATHER

☐ Hot ☐ Mild ☐ Cold BM Pressure: ______

☐ Dry ☐ Humid ☐ Wet Allergen Levels: ______

☐ Sunny ☐ Cloudy

STRESS LEVELS

None	Low	Medium	High	Max	@$#%!

FOOD / DRINKS + NON-RELIEF MEDICATION / SUPPLEMENTS

item / meal	*time*	*meds / supplements*	*dose*	*time*

How many drinks?

water	⇨	① ② ③ ④ ⑤ ⑥ ⑦ ⑧ ⑨ ⑩
caffeine	⇨	① ② ③ ④ ⑤ ⑥ ⑦ ⑧ ⑨ ⑩
alcohol	⇨	① ② ③ ④ ⑤ ⑥ ⑦ ⑧ ⑨ ⑩

HORMONES

☐ Menstruating ☐ Menopause ☐ PMS ☐ N/A | other

COMPUTER USE / READING

☐ None ☐ Some ☐ A lot Total time:

☐ Sitting ☐ Standing ☐ Mixture Breaks every:

PHYSICAL ACTIVITY

☐ None ☐ Minimal ☐ Some ☐ Sweatin' ☐ I'm beat

DETAILS: ______________________________

RELIEF MEASURES

☐ Medication ☐ Massage ☐ Sleep ☐ Exercise

☐ Water ☐ Cold/Ice ☐ Heat/Bath ☐ Other

DETAILS: ______________________________

DID IT WORK? ☐ Nope ☐ A bit ☐ Mostly ☐ 100%

Notes

Additional Notes

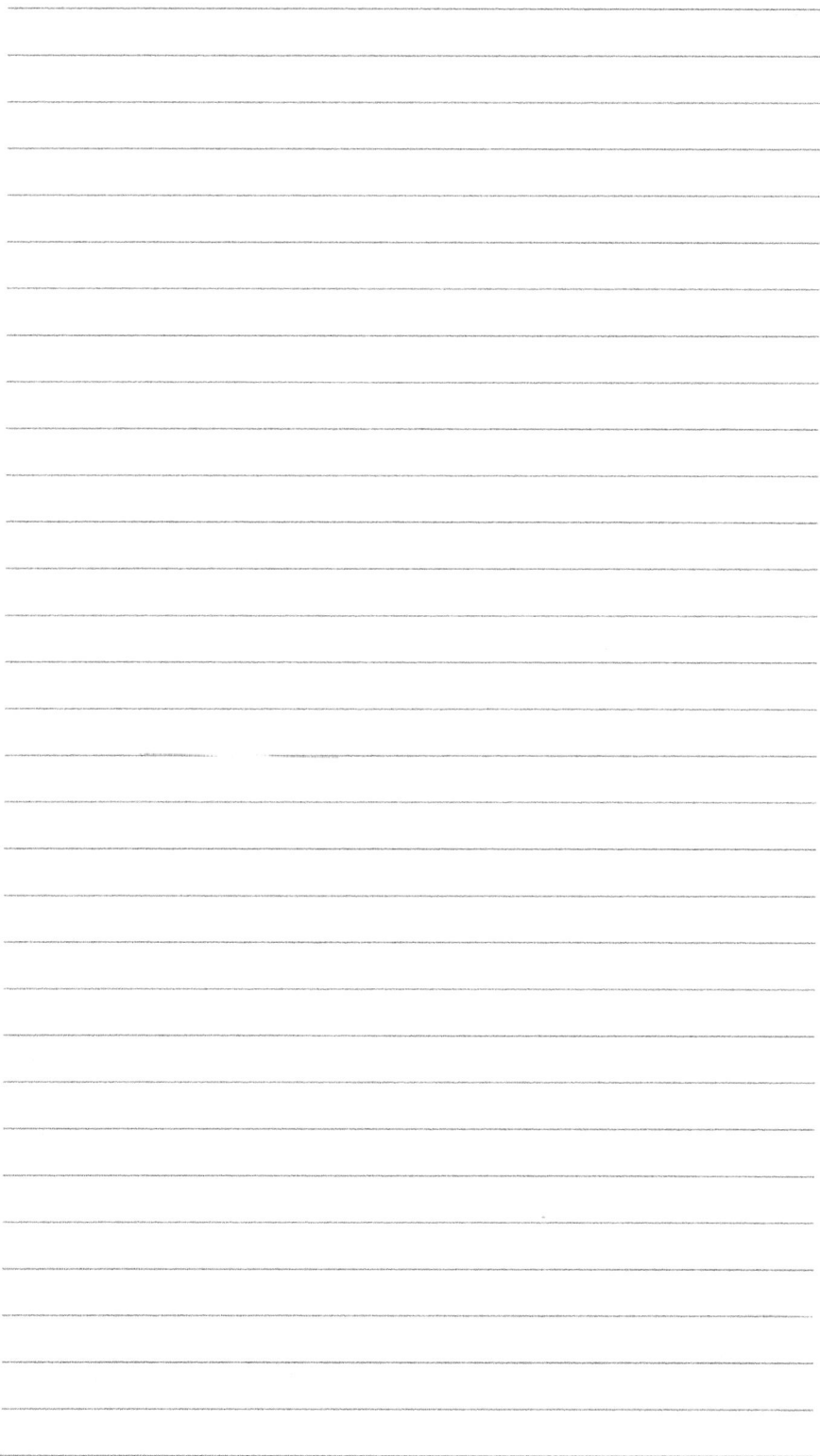

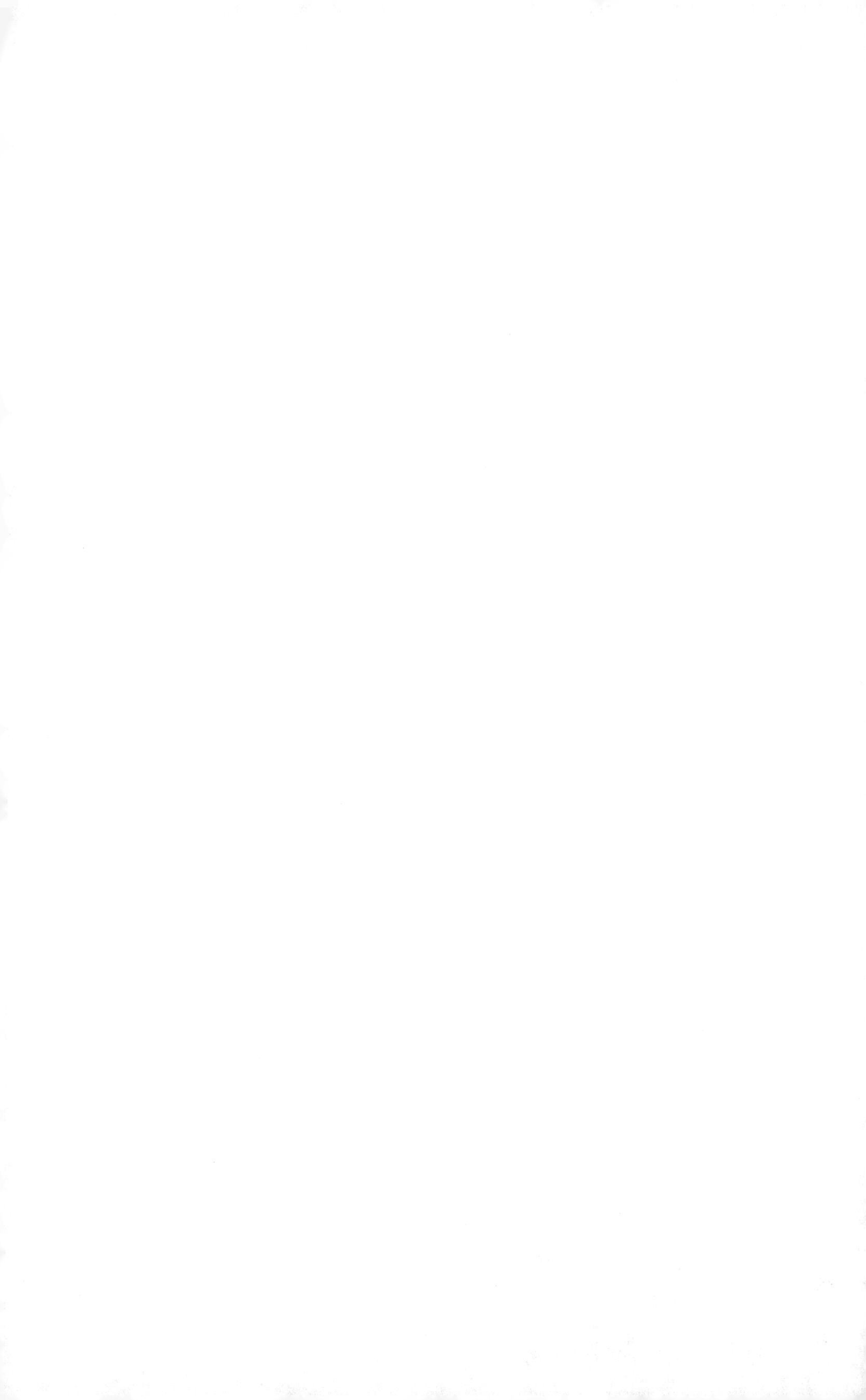

www.ingramcontent.com/pod-product-compliance
Lightning Source LLC
Chambersburg PA
CBHW070123030426
42335CB00016B/2247

9781990271243